CANCER ETIOLOGY, DIAGNOSIS AND TREATMENTS

EPENDYMOMAS

PROGNOSTIC FACTORS, TREATMENT STRATEGIES AND CLINICAL OUTCOMES

CANCER ETIOLOGY, DIAGNOSIS AND TREATMENTS

Additional books in this series can be found on Nova's website under the Series tab.

Additional e-books in this series can be found on Nova's website under the e-book tab.

CANCER ETIOLOGY, DIAGNOSIS AND TREATMENTS

EPENDYMOMAS

PROGNOSTIC FACTORS, TREATMENT STRATEGIES AND CLINICAL OUTCOMES

RAQUEL FOWLER
EDITOR

NOVA BIOMEDICAL
New York

NOTICE TO THE READER

The Publisher has taken reasonable care in the preparation of this book, but makes no expressed or implied warranty of any kind and assumes no responsibility for any errors or omissions. No liability is assumed for incidental or consequential damages in connection with or arising out of information contained in this book. The Publisher shall not be liable for any special, consequential, or exemplary damages resulting, in whole or in part, from the readers' use of, or reliance upon, this material. Any parts of this book based on government reports are so indicated and copyright is claimed for those parts to the extent applicable to compilations of such works.

Independent verification should be sought for any data, advice or recommendations contained in this book. In addition, no responsibility is assumed by the publisher for any injury and/or damage to persons or property arising from any methods, products, instructions, ideas or otherwise contained in this publication.

This publication is designed to provide accurate and authoritative information with regard to the subject matter covered herein. It is sold with the clear understanding that the Publisher is not engaged in rendering legal or any other professional services. If legal or any other expert assistance is required, the services of a competent person should be sought. FROM A DECLARATION OF PARTICIPANTS JOINTLY ADOPTED BY A COMMITTEE OF THE AMERICAN BAR ASSOCIATION AND A COMMITTEE OF PUBLISHERS.

Additional color graphics may be available in the e-book version of this book.

Library of Congress Cataloging-in-Publication Data

ISBN: 978-1-63484-405-5

Library of Congress Control Number: 2015959364

Published by Nova Science Publishers, Inc. † New York

CONTENTS

PREFACE

This book provides research on ependymomas, a rare brain tumor that arises from the ependymal cells of the intra-ventricular central nervous system (CNS) parenchyma with a propensity to affect both children and adults. Ependymomas account for only 1.9% of all primary brain and CNS tumors.

Chapter 1 - Prognosis plays a pivotal role in the treatment a patient receives and how aggressively treatment is pursued. It also helps give the patient a sense of how well those in similar clinical situations have fared over the course of their treatment. However, with ependymomas, the struggle to provide consistent markers of prognostication has proven especially difficult. This is largely due to the difficulty in establishing a cohesive patient population for review due to the rarity of this tumor entity. In fact ependymomas constitute just 1.9% of all primary brain and central nervous system tumors according to the latest Central Brain Tumor Registry of the United States (CBTRUS) statistical report. With relative histological heterogeneity within a single tumor, patients may not always fit neatly into a specific WHO classification. Furthermore, histology may have varying prognostic significance depending upon tumor location. More recent discoveries have also indicated molecular diversity amongst ependymomas that may help explain different responses to treatment and outcomes. With relatively limited knowledge of the role different aspects of ependymoma histological and molecular pathology, clinical course and treatment play on outcome, the authors plan to discuss current knowledge in this field and highlight future directions of research that might help their better understand this rare tumor entity.

Chapter 2 - *Background and Purpose.* Ependymoma is a rare primary brain tumor that arises from the ependymal cells of the intra-ventricular central nervous system (CNS) parenchyma with a propensity to affect both children and adults. This study aims to investigate the effects of gender, age, race, tumor grade, and treatment on clinical outcomes of ependymoma diagnosed patients.

Methods. Retrospective clinical analysis of ependymoma and systematic review of histological data were included in this study from the Scott and White Brain Tumor Registry collected from 1976-2013.

Results. About 30% of pediatric ependymomas were diagnosed in children younger than three years of age. Patients with completely resected tumors have an estimated 5-year survival rate of 67-80%, compared to an estimated 5-year survival rate of 22-47% in patients with incompletely resected tumors. Patients treated with post-operative radiation have a better outcome than patients who do not receive a radiation. Focal radiation to the site of the tumor lowers the risk of tumor recurrence at the site of origin. Ependymoma recurrence was observed in patients with grade III and II tumors. Ependymomas rarely metastasize outside of the CNS.

Most patients who deceased after treatment were under the age of 25. Pediatric 5-year survival rate was approximately 66% compared with the adult 5-year survival rate which was 78%. The 5-year male and female survival rates were in average of 80% and 60%, respectively. The 5-year survival rates of the White patients and patients of all other ethnicities as a single group were 73% and 75%, respectively. Patients with primary tumor sites in brain stem, frontal lobe, and parietal lobe have an excellent overall survival and low risk of tumor recurrence.

Conclusion. This study exhibits that surgical treatment with attempted gross total resection is a gold standard in treatment of ependymoma. The extent of surgical resection, age, and amount of tumor remaining after surgery are the primary factors influencing survival. Primary tumor site is another important prognostic factor for evaluation of short and long-term outcomes of ependymoma. Radiation therapy requires more future studies in order to elucidate more definitive treatment guidelines.

Chapter 3 - Anaplastic ependymoma represents a nosographic and epidemiological problem as it has been, and still it is, difficult to distinguish from grade II tumors, and thus its incidence cannot be exactly calculated. The main features required for the tumor recognition are high cell density, high number of mitoses or high Ki-67/MIB-1 labeling index. However, the crucial point is represented by the threshold of the number of mitoses, which in the authors' experience, must exceed 20%.

A true genetic marker for the anaplastic variant is still lacking; however, a small spectrum of genetic aberrations is usually found.

The differential diagnosis of the anaplastic variant *versus* neuroepithelial tumors is not problematic. The only diagnostic critical point is represented by the appearance of anaplasia in *foci* that can escape detection or of an advanced status of anaplasia that hampers the recognition of the tumor as ependymomatous.

In this chapter, prognosis, prognostic factors and survival will be discussed, taking into account that the tumor may have four different locations and may need different surgical treatments. The standard strategy relies on radiation therapy while chemotherapy plays a secondary role. Temozolomide and other drugs are currently employed in clinical trials.

Chapter 4 - Background: Intraspinal ependymomas (ISE) constitute approximately 60% of all intradural spinal tumors; around 50% are intramedullary ependymoma (IME) and the remaining myxopapillary ependymoma (MPE).

Methods: This chapter contains a contemporary review of the literature and an evidence-based systematic review about ISE. A published case series of the University of Wisconsin Hospital (UWH), of patients operated upon for ISE, was also presented to illustrate this manuscript. All this information was properly discussed in order to propose guidelines for the management of patients with ISE.

Results: This chapter was written based on the review of many relevant and updated scientific sources, including the author's evidence-based systematic review about ISE, based on 27 papers (1,211 patients). A review of series regarding IME was based on 4 papers (143 patients). The overall recurrence/progression rate was 3.63%. The highest incidence of recurrence occurred in patients submitted to subtotal resection (STR) alone (5.26%), followed by GTR alone (3.37%). The review regarding MPE was based on 5 papers (199 patients). The overall recurrence/progression rate was 24.12%. Gross-total resection (GTR) alone resulted in 15.21% of recurrence, while GTR plus radiotherapy (XRT) reduced the recurrence rate to 5.26%. The published UWH case series of 38 patients was also described. Nineteen patients were operated for IME. GTR was achieved in 11, being 4 *en bloc* GTR, 6 piecemeal, not specified in 1 case, and all remained disease-free. STR was accomplished in 6 patients, 3 were living with stable disease; 2 with progression of the neoplasm, and 1 died after the tumor progression. Partial removal was performed in 2 patients, they were submitted to XRT, 1 deceased, and another was living with stable tumor. Eleven were disease-free, and 8 had tumor recurrence, progression and/or stable disease. Nineteen patients had MPE. GTR was achieved in 14, seven *en bloc* GTR, all remained disease-free, 7 piecemeal GTR, and 2 cases had tumor recurrence. STR was accomplished in 2, they were submitted to XRT, and they were living with stable disease. Partial resection was performed in 2, they were re-operated and submitted to XRT, and were living with the neoplasm. Biopsy was performed in 1 patient. Thirteen patients remained disease-free and 6 had tumor recurrence, progression and/or stable disease.

Conclusions: This manuscript was based on level IV of medical evidence (recommendation grade C) supporting that early diagnosis and better preoperative neurological status can improve the postoperative neurological outcome in patients treated with ISE; supporting the role of GTR; supporting postoperative XRT to reduce the recurrence/progression of the tumor in patients with ISE submitted to incomplete resection; and also supporting the use of routine postoperative XRT to potentially reduce the recurrence/progression of the tumor in patients operated for MPE, even after GTR. Intraspinal ependymoma is not as "benign" as proposed by its histology, but has a high potential of recurrence and/or progression. In this chapter the authors describe the clinical symptoms of intramedullary tumors and their neuroradiological features, provide a description of modern surgical techniques, and discuss the postoperative results and outcomes on the basis of UWH series and the evidence-based systematic review of the literature.

Chapter 5 - The vast majority of ependymal neoplasms appear to arise in a sporadic fashion. There are, however, subsets of these neoplasms that are known to be associated with hereditary tumor syndromes or neurocutaneous disorders. The most recognized of these associations is the predisposition of Neurofibromatosis Type II (NF2) patients toward the development of certain nervous system tumors including ependymomas, vestibular and schwannomas, and meningiomas. NF2 gene mutations (chromosome 22q12.2) are well-recognized features of these patients and their tumors. Less commonly, ependymomas have been reported in patients with MEN 1 syndrome, which is characterized by the development of multiple endocrine neoplasms. The MEN 1 gene (chromosome 11q13) is involved in allelic losses and rearrangements in ependymomas. Ependymomas have also been described rarely in patients with Turcot syndrome (MSH2 gene on chromosome 2p22-p21). Anecdotal cases of ependymoma have also been described in association with disorders such as Li-Fraumeni syndrome, Neurofibromatosis Type I, Cowden syndrome, von Hippel-Lindau syndrome and Tuberous Sclerosis. This chapter reviews the literature on ependymal neoplasms arising in the setting of hereditary tumor syndromes.

Chapter 6 - Ependymomas are the third commonest tumor of the central nervous system (CNS) accounting for 6-12% of brain tumors in children. Even with advances in neurosurgical, neuroimaging and postoperative adjuvant therapy, the prognosis remains poor with a 5 year progression free survival (PFS) of 23-45%. Recurrence of tumor develops in

50% of cases, even after complete surgical resection followed by radiotherapy. To-date no chemotherapeutic regimen has proven to be of significant clinical benefit. Predicting tumor behavior and defining robust correlates of disease outcome based on histopathology and clinical characteristics remains suboptimal. Paucity of cell lines, failure to develop animal models of these tumors unlike other CNS malignancies, has precluded better understanding of the oncogenic drivers, undermining development of targeted therapy. Thus these tumors have remained therapeutically frustrating and enigmatic. However, over the last few years major breakthrough in the understanding of the molecular biology and subtypes, cellular origin of these tumor cells and signaling pathways are now providing insights into development of biological targeted therapies in ependymoma. It is now clear that even with histopathological similarities, these are genetically heterogeneous tumors with diverse clinical outcomes. Rapid evolution of data now suggests three principal molecular subgroups of ependymomas in children, based on gene clustering. These include supratentorial (ST), posterior fossa (PF) and the spinal (SP) and posterior fossa (PF) subtypes. More recently based on transcriptome profiling, two subgroups (Group A and B) of PF ependymomas have been identified with distinct molecular, clinical characteristics and specific chromosomal aberrations. Signaling pathways specific to these subtypes have now been delineated, raising hopes of defining therapeutic targets. In the years ahead sustained research endeavors are needed to enhance the authors' understanding of the elusive biology of these tumors. This will enable the authors to profile optimal biologically driven targeted therapy in addition to conventional treatment modalities to improve survival rate.

In: Ependymomas
Editor: Raquel Fowler

ISBN: 978-1-63484-405-5

Chapter 1

PROGNOSIS AND OUTCOMES IN EPENDYMAL TUMORS

Nicholas R. Metrus[1,*], MD, and David Cachia[2], MD
[1]The University of Texas MD Anderson Cancer Center,
Department of Neuro-Oncology, Houston, TX, US
The University of Texas Medical Branch,
Department of Neurology, Galveston, TX, US
[2]Medical University of South Carolina, Department of Neurosurgery, US

ABSTRACT

Prognosis plays a pivotal role in the treatment a patient receives and how aggressively treatment is pursued. It also helps give the patient a sense of how well those in similar clinical situations have fared over the course of their treatment. However, with ependymomas, the struggle to provide consistent markers of prognostication has proven especially difficult. This is largely due to the difficulty in establishing a cohesive patient population for review due to the rarity of this tumor entity. In fact ependymomas constitute just 1.9% of all primary brain and central nervous system tumors according to the latest Central Brain Tumor Registry of the United States (CBTRUS) statistical report. With relative histological heterogeneity within a single tumor, patients may not always fit neatly into a specific WHO classification. Furthermore, histology may have varying prognostic significance depending upon tumor location. More recent discoveries have also indicated molecular diversity amongst ependymomas that may help explain different responses to treatment and outcomes. With relatively limited knowledge of the role different aspects of ependymoma histological and molecular pathology, clinical course and treatment play on outcome, we plan to discuss current knowledge in this field and highlight future directions of research that might help us better understand this rare tumor entity.

* Phone: 409-772-8058 Fax: 409-772-6940 Email: nrmetrus@utmb.edu.

Introduction

Ependymomas account for only 1.9% of all primary brain and central nervous system (CNS) tumors. In view of their uncommon occurrence, there is limited literature available, compared to more common tumors. Of the studies that do exist, many are retrospective and span over decades in order to incorporate an adequate sample size to draw any conclusions. This in itself limits the significance of the findings. Furthermore, many of the studies are conducted out of single institutions making generalization of the findings problematic. With these limitations in mind, we summarize the prognostic features thought to impact outcome in ependymomas.

Histology/Pathology

Ependymal tumors are histologically classified under the World Health Organization (WHO) classification as follows: myxopapillary and subependymomas fall under grade I, ependymomas (further subclassified into papillary, clear cell or tanycytic) are grade II and anaplastic ependymomas are grade III.

Grade I tumors tend not to be infiltrative into surrounding normal brain or spinal cord parenchyma which distinguishes them from grade II and III tumors. By virtue of this biologic distinction, they are more amenable to complete resection and rarely ever exhibit malignant transformation into a higher-grade tumor. Grade I tumors are therefore potentially curable. Grade II are less likely to allow for complete resection by virtue of their infiltrative nature, and grade III even more so. Even with extensive resection, the rate of cure is lower in grade II ependymal tumors. They, unlike the aforementioned grade I tumor, can have the potential to transform into grade III tumors. Grade III ependymomas, though less infiltrative into surrounding normal parenchyma than malignant astrocytomas, are almost never cured with surgical resection and frequently recur [1].

On gross pathology, in the fourth ventricle (the most common cerebral site for ependymomas), the tumor has a grayish pink appearance, is firm and cauliflower-like. Those in the cerebrum may arise from the wall of the lateral ventricle and be significantly larger in size, growing into the lateral ventricle and becoming up to several centimeters in diameter. They tend to be more clearly demarcated from the surrounding normal tissue than an astrocytoma which is traditionally more infiltrative. However, they are not encapsulated. Under the microscope, the cells of an ependymoma form rosettes with central lumens in some cases, but more often will form circular arrangements around blood vessels or "pseudorosettes". Epithelial ependymomas may appear more densely cellular and anaplastic ependymomas will exhibit high mitotic activity, nuclear atypia, necrosis and endothelial proliferation [2].

Per Metellus et al. there are four distinguishable classes of pathological misdiagnoses when it comes to ependymal tumors [3]. The first is erroneous diagnoses, when ependymomas are confused with, and subsequently misdiagnosed as another tumor such as a neurocytoma, medulloblastoma, metastatic carcinoma or papillary meningioma. The second class is the inability to distinguish an ependymoma from a subependymoma. The third, results from the more recent discovery of new pathological entities that can be confused with ependymal tumors and include papillary tumors of the pineal region, glioneuronal tumors and oligodendrogliomas with neurocytic differentiation. The final class is gliomas frequently misdiagnosed as ependymomas. A postulation within the same paper was that since *olig2* staining is most often missing in ependymomas, it has the potential to be a means of ruling out ependymomas when faced with a concern of ependymoma vs. other glioma. These errors make accurate evaluation of prognosis and outcomes of this already rare tumor more difficult.

This is further complicated by the lack of strict criteria on how to histologically define anaplasia in ependymomas that has led to varied conclusions as to whether or not histology is important in impacting outcomes in ependymomas. While WHO grade correlates with a better overall survival as well as better progression free survival in a univariate analysis, Metellus et al. proposed the use of the Marseille grading system; an alternate grading system [3]. This grading system consists of only three criteria: necrosis, whether or not microvascular proliferation was present, and mitotic index. When using this grading system, they found that the ependymomas that exhibited a criterion of 0 or 1 had a significantly better prognosis than ependymomas with 2 or 3 of these histological criteria. Furthermore, when they compared this grading system to the WHO classification, they found that the Marseille grading system was the only one of the two to have significant correlation with overall survival and progression free survival in multivariate analysis.

Upon close inspection of the methodology of some series on ependymomas, a lack of a central pathology review may contribute to the ultimate conclusions drawn from the data of the series. For example, in a paper by Reni et al. they concluded that histological grade did not have a statically significant correlation with survival [4] However, they did not use central pathological review for their subjects and thus relied on pathologists who may have been inconsistent in defining "anaplasia" during their tissue analyses [3]. Also, there are a number of primary CNS tumors that are very similar in appearance to ependymomas which can make consistency amongst diagnoses difficult. In one example, some series that used central review of putative ependymomas found that almost 30% were actually misdiagnosed [5]. In another example from MD Anderson Cancer Center, 18 additional study participants were able to be recruited into a study about adult ependymal tumor prognosis when, upon central review, their tumors which were previously diagnosed as something other than ependymoma were subsequently reclassified as such [6].

Molecular Markers

The role of molecular markers in predicting outcomes in ependymomas is a much more novel field than those of surgical resection, histology, age, etc. As such most of the data has only been published over the last few years. Some of the more recent data is suggestive of ependymomas exhibiting biological characteristics that differ based on their anatomic location, ie cerebral vs infratentorial vs spinal cord. In intracranial ependymomas specifically, there is a high expression of members of the NOTCH as well as the Sonic Hedgehog pathway. In spinal ependymomas, there is more expression of Homeobox containing (HOX) family genes [7].

In a study by Wani et al. which focused specifically on infratentorial ependymomas, unsupervised clustering of available gene expression microarray data was used in order to create two subgroups of tumors based on expression of genes associated with mesenchyme [8]. PCR was run on the genes defining each subgroup. The end result was a 10 gene prognostic signature that served as an independent predictor of recurrence free survival, once it had been adjusted for clinical factors. Analysis of the known functions of those genes incorporated into the 10 gene signature showed that a poor survival was associated with increased expression of genes associated with angiogenesis, extracellular matrix and proliferation.

There are a number of other prognostic markers that have been studied. One of those is Ki-67, which is an immunolabelling index that has been found to be useful as a prognostic indicator in ependymomas of the posterior fossa in pediatric patients. One study proposed that the Ki-67 labeling index be used during trials of novel adjunctive therapies as part of the histological evaluation [9]. However, one of the downfalls of Ki-67 labeling index is that, due to its large variance in values, it may be problematic to use it as a means of separating tumors with significantly different biological behaviors. Another potential prognostic marker is the gene survivin whose expression is plentiful in mammalian embryonic development and which plays a role in inhibition of cell death and as regulation of the mitotic spindle checkpoint [10]. Previous studies had noted that survivin expression in many different tumors was, more often than not, a poor prognostic sign. However, it had also been noted that it was an independent variable for a favorable prognosis in two large clinical studies on breast and gastric carcinomas. Using samples of perinatal and pediatric autopsy cases, tissue analysis showed that survivin was heavily expressed in both the choroid plexus as well as the normal ependyma. Expression of the nuclear form of survivin had a correlation with morphologic tumor grade where loss of nuclear expression was associated with progressive cytologic anaplasia, suggesting that abnormally low levels of survivin expression could be used as a marker for more progressive disease. Another study, using multivariate analysis, found that low expression of the protein nucleolin was independently associated with a more favorable prognosis in pediatric ependymomas [11]. Also of note, the same study found that the aforementioned survivin and Ki-67 correlated with histological grade, but not with outcome.

Studies have found that ependymomas with chromosomal gain of 1q and/or homozygous deletion of CDKN2A have predominantly anaplastic histology and poor prognosis. The homozygous deletion of CDKN2A is particularly indicative of aggressive clinical behavior as well as metastatic spread. On the other hand, patients with ependymomas who had chromosomal gain of 9, 15q and 18 or loss of chromosome 6 had excellent outcomes with current treatment regimens [12].

Most recently, focus has shifted to the analysis of DNA methylation. The DNA methylation patterns in tumors have stability in molecular memory of their respective cell origins which remains evident throughout the course of the disease. This feature makes DNA methylation patterns a reliable means for tumor classification. One study aimed to use DNA methylation profiling to establish a uniform molecular classification [13]. The end result was a collection of nine molecular subgroups that encompassed all age groups, addressed each of three anatomical compartments (spine, posterior fossa and supratentorial) and proved each group to be distinct one from the other. The analysis was performed by using only a very small amount of DNA material and thus would be ideal for a method adopted as a routine clinical application. In fact, the DNA methylation marks are so durable, they can be recovered even after a tumor sample has been stored for years in formalin fixed paraffin embedded tissue or in frozen tumor samples with RNA degradation [14]. Similar to medulloblastoma, the molecular subgrouping of ependymomas remains stable throughout the course of the disease, thought to be because DNA methylation profiles reflect their epigenetic memory cell of origin. The study found that when they applied their method of molecular classification, most of the ependymomas in high-risk patients (mostly children) for which therapeutic options have shown dismal outcomes fell into just two of the nine molecular subgroups that were identified. These were the posterior fossa anaplastic ependymomas and the supratentorial ependymomas positive for the "RELA fusion"; a chromothripsis (chromosome shattering event) of chromosome 11 which results in a fusion of RELA (the principal effector for NFκB signaling in 70% of supratentorial tumors but not those of the posterior fossa or spinal cord) [15] and poorly characterized C11orf95.

Another recent study classified ependymomas into five molecularly distinct ependymoma subtypes by location: C11orf95-RELA positive and C11orf95-RELA negative tumors of the supratentorial compartment, CIMP (CPG Island Methylator Phenotype) positive and CIMP negative tumors of the posterior fossa, and spinal cord tumors [16]. Each subtype was distinct to its region of origin. Initially, the genome was broken down for analysis of single nucleotide variations, insertions or focal (defined as <5 gene) copy number variations. However, few of those existed in ependymomas. Instead, investigators found that there were several structural variations, specifically on chromosome 11q12.1-q13.3 which caused a translocation of C11orf95 and RELA. They additionally found that tumors that were C11orf95-RELA positive also expressed increased amounts of CCND1 which is a direct transcriptional target of NFκB signaling, as well as L1CAM which serves the functions of cell-cell adhesion, invasion and for NFκB activation in tumors.

A different team analyzed 47 hindbrain ependymomas with whole-genome and whole-exome sequencing, concluding that while genetically bland (low mutation rate, no significant recurrent somatic single nucleotide variants) they all exhibited a CpG Island melthylator (CIMP) phenotype, defined as tumors having more methylated CpG sites, more genes with significant CpG methylation and more genes that are transcriptionally silenced by CpG hypermethylation. CpG methylation drives a transcriptional silencing that converges exclusively on targets of the Polycomb repressive complex 2 which represses expression of differentiation genes through trimethylation of H3K27. Thus tumors exhibiting the CIMP phenotype were shown to be responsive to clinical drugs which used DNA or H3K27 methylation as targets. Response was demonstrated both *in vitro* and *in vivo* [17]. The advantage of molecularly understanding the basis of these tumors, is that this might eventually lead to drugable targets. One high-throughput drug screen was developed as a conglomeration of 3,161 bioactive compounds, 1,648 "orphan-kinase inhibitor scaffolds", 367 specific kinase inhibitors and 275 FDA approved drugs. The result was that of the 5,303 total compounds, 140 of them displayed anti-ependymoma activity. One such compound is the well-known chemotherapeutic agent, 5-fluorouracil which was shown to be effective against the highly sensitive supratentorial C11orf95-RELA fusion-negative tumors [18]. These molecular classifications can in the near future be included with the current standard of histopathological classification.

Anatomical Location

The incidence of ependymomas across the CNS differs by age. In fact whilst in children the most common location is an infratentorial origin (54%) followed by supratentorial (32%) and spinal cord (11%) location, in adults ependymomas typically arise in the spinal cord (64%), followed by infratentorial (24%) and supratentorial location (11%) [19]. One study of 238 WHO Grade II and III ependymomas found that the histology of the tumor varied based on its anatomical location and that when the specific histological attributes of a tumor were taken into consideration as related to the anatomical location, outcomes varied among these tumors [20]. If an ependymoma was in the posterior fossa and exhibited histologic evidence of hypercellular areas, necrosis, microvascular proliferation or elevated mitotic rate, there was a worse progression free survival. Tumors in the same location which exhibited extensive ependymal canal formation had no association with progression free survival. Supratentorial ependymomas with histology showing microvascular proliferation, elevated mitotic rate, or extensive canal formation had a worse progression free survival. However, the histology of hypercellular areas and necrosis did not have an association with progression free survival, if that tumor was located supratentorially. In the spinal cord, all histological variants had no association with progression free survival. The study makes a strong case for a more site-specific grading criteria incorporated into future classification systems.

Surgical Resection

Currently, surgical resection is the first step in standard of care treatment. As ependymomas tend to grow into ventricles, commonly, patients initially present with signs and symptoms of increased intracranial pressure. Usually arising from the fourth ventricle, cerebral ependymomas can extend through the foramen of Luschka and Magendie and may later invade the medulla. These patients may present with symptoms of nausea, vomiting, vertigo, neck flexion or head tilt. The symptoms have also been described as similar to the presentation of a medulloblastoma but with a more protracted time course and lacking early cerebellar signs [2]. Generally the symptoms are non-specific which is why generalized symptoms may go on for a while without neurologic workup, thus delaying time to diagnosis of tumor. Interval between the first symptom and diagnosis can range from weeks, in the most malignant tumor types, to years in lower grade ependymomas.

Maximal surgical resection when safe to perform, is the standard of care for all ependymoma patients. Gross total resection (GTR) has been shown to be associated with improved outcomes in most studies [3, 21, 22, 23]. However, getting a true complete resection is often difficult with reported success rates ranging from 25%-93% in cases of supratentorial ependymomas and 5% to 72% in infratentorial ependymomas. Within the intratentorial location the possibility of obtaining a GTR depends upon their specific location of origin. For example, gross total resection can be achieved in up to 100% of cases when the tumor sits in the roof of the fourth ventricle, 86% when within the mid-ventricle and 54% when located in the lateral recesses. In terms of spinal cord tumors, most are low grade and thus it is easier to achieve a complete resection by virtue of less infiltration of the surrounding tissue. In spinal tumors, a reported 27%-45% of cases were removed with no functional impairment [4]. Post-operative imaging will help to analyze the extent of resection, and further resection is encouraged if residual tumor is found [3]. In cases of recurrence, surgical resection is recommended as the first consideration for re-treatment [24].

While favored as a treatment of choice for ependymomas, surgical resection is obviously not without its own risks. Some intracranial tumor locations are not amenable to resection, such as intrinsic brainstem tumors, or those adhering to cranial nerves or vascular structures. In the case of spinal cord ependymomas, like myxopapillary tumors, there is a risk of rupturing the tumor capsule and thus causing dissemination of tumor cells into the surrounding CSF [1]. CSF dissemination is almost always fatal. In the event of CSF dissemination, early detection and post-operative craniospinal radiation in combination with chemotherapy gives the patient the best chance of survival [25]. For intracranial ependymomas, where incidence of dissemination is approximately 15% and is more common with posterior fossa tumors and anaplastic ependymomas, analysis of CSF for dissemination too early after tumor resection can be misleading. Therefore it is recommended that CSF analysis be postponed for at least two weeks following resection. Outside of this two-week post-operative guideline, surveillance frequency for CSF dissemination has not been well established. Incidence of dissemination remains relatively low, but since early diagnosis may impact treatment options and outcomes, there should be a low threshold to perform CSF analysis on patients in follow up after resection if there is clinical suspicion for dissemination [1].

Age

Age of the patient plays a significant role in prognostication for several reasons. As described above the anatomical distribution of ependymal tumors varies among different age groups. Additional considerations based on age are also made when deciding treatment options. A study by the Pediatric Oncology Group looked specifically at ependymomas in a patient population with ages less than three years old [26]. They broke down the patient population into two groups; 0-23 months at diagnosis (who received chemotherapy with alternating cycles of vincristine + cyclophosphamide and cisplatin + etoposide for two years followed by radiation) and 24-36 months at diagnosis (who received the same chemotherapy for just one year followed by radiation). They found that the second group had a much better five-year survival rate (63.3% vs 25.7%). It was determined that the most likely reason for the difference in survival was the difference in delay to radiation (one year in comparison to two years), prompting them to recommend that radiation not be delayed greater than one year in treatment of ependymoma. This goes against what is recommended in other CNS malignancies where radiation is delayed at least beyond 3 years of age in view of the impact of radiation on neurocognitive development. The alternative hypothesis was that ependymomas in younger children have a more aggressive biology. Consensus remains that, in general, the younger the child the worse the prognosis [27].

On the opposite end of the age spectrum, few studies have been done on the subject of ependymal tumors in an older patient population. One study, believed to be the first of its kind with a focus strictly on ependymomas in patients age 60 and up at time of diagnosis, demonstrated that the tumor location, tumor histology and surgical margin may be key predictors of outcome in older ependymoma patients [28]. The study looked at 367 cases, mostly low grade with only 19 anaplastic tumors. They found that the patients' overall mortality risk and ependymoma-specific mortality risk were similar. However, tumor histology was a significant predictor of cause specific, but not overall, mortality hazard. In addition, the notion that better outcome is associated with gross total resection holds true for the >60 year old population but the older a patient is, the less likely they are to pursue and ultimately receive aggressive cancer therapies.

Recurrence

Recurrence is seen in a significant number of patients with both spinal and cranial ependymomas. The dominant pattern of recurrence is local failure. The initial step should be restaging of the tumor including craniospinal MRI, even for intracranial ependymomas as leptomeningeal dissemination has been reported in 10% of cases of low grade ependymomas and 30% of cases with high grade ependymomas [24]. Initial consideration should be gross total resection when possible [24]. Based on the findings of a series by Chowdhary et al. a 39% 2 year survival was achieved in a cohort of patients where 90% got surgery at the time of relapse [29]. However, when the recurrence is inoperable, and the patient has not had previous radiation, consensus is to use radiation. Even in cases where the patient has been previously irradiated, radiosurgery to small lesions or external beam radiotherapy to small lesions could be considered [24].

Armstrong et al. evaluated 123 adults with ependymal tumors with a breakdown of 40 brain, 80 spine and 3 brain and spine tumors [6]. Of those, 108 were low grade and 15 were anaplastic. The results of the study, with a average follow up of 5.5 years was that patient's with spinal ependymomas had a median time of 25 months to their first recurrence and 20 months to their second recurrence. Of those with intracranial ependymomas, the median time to first recurrence was 21 months and 10.5 months to second recurrence. When grade III lesions were analyzed on their own, median time to first recurrence was significantly less at 18 months and 12 months to second. Median survival could not be calculated for spine ependymomas in the study. For brain ependymomas, those with low-grade tumors had a medial survival rate of 221 months while those with anaplastic tumors had a median survival of 67 months.

One study that directly addresses the issue of recurrence of ependymomas in the pediatric population is by Bouffet et al. who successfully re-irradiated 18 pediatric ependymomas with no severe acute complications and obtained a survival rate of 81% at three years [30]. The study also made a significant additional finding; that the time to the next recurrence was longer after the second irradiation than it had been from first irradiation to first recurrence. Extension of the time to relapse after second dose of irradiation suggested that there was a mechanism of hypersensitization, or a cumulative toxicity, of the ependymoma cells to the second dose. Supporting this finding was the observation that patients who did not receive radiation initially and received radiation at recurrence did not have as favorable of an outcome as those who received radiation both initially and at recurrence. In an attempt to better understand this phenomenon, expression of a marker of continuous DNA damage, γH2AX, was measured and a correlation was found between high expression and sensitivity to reirradiation, suggesting that there is a mechanism of persistent DNA damage that overwhelms the cellular repair machinery leading to cell death. When recurrence is evaluated, it is important to evaluate whether the study follow up period was long enough to make significant conclusions. Whitaker et al. concluded in 1991 that the 10-year progression free survival rate for spinal ependymomas was 68% [31]. However, the study only had a follow up period of 70 months. A more recent study by Gomez et al. in 2005 extended the follow up period to 121 months and found that the length of follow up had a significant impact on the amount of documented recurrence [32]. In that study of 37 patients, who all received resection and postoperative radiation, 21 of the 37 had recurrence and of the 21 with recurrence, 12 of those occurred at least five years later. Because of the extended time for follow up, they found local relapse rates were higher than previously reported in the literature since the recurrences tended to be outside the previously established follow up intervals. The study found that the percentage of five, ten and fifteen year progression free patients was 75% ± 7.4%, 50% ± 9.1% and 46% ± 9.3%, respectively. The median time to progression in the study was 68 months with a range of 2 to 324 months.

CONCLUSION

Prognosticating outcome in ependymal tumors remains fraught with difficulty for the clinician. The rarity of the tumors, retrospective nature of the studies and inconsistent interpretation of the histologic/pathologic diagnosis amongst pathologists limits the data available in comparison to other CNS tumors that are more common. One of the least controversial prognostic factors is extent of surgical resection though the degree of benefit varies amongst studies. There is more debate amongst the other factors that may (or in some cases it is argued, may *not*) play a role in patient prognosis including tumor location, recurrence rates, age of the patient, or tumor histology.

One of the more rapidly evolving literature topics in ependymomas is the examination of the tumors at the genetic level. It is now becoming clearer that these tumors have varying histology and genetic makeup dependent upon whether they are located above the tentorium, within the posterior fossa or within the spinal cord. New developments in ependymal tumor research are now focusing on the distinct genetic makeup of these tumors to provide more specific targeted therapies. This genetic information and classification may one day also supersede the current histological classification. It is only by understanding the biology of these tumors that we can make strides in accurately diagnosing, managing, treating and predicting outcomes of these rare tumors.

REFERENCES

[1] Gilbert, MR; Ruda, R; Soffietti, R. Ependymomas in adults. *Curr. Neurol. Neurosci. Rep.* 2010 10, 240-247.

[2] Ropper, AH; Samuels, MA; Klein, JP. Adams and Victor's Principles of Neurology. Tenth Edition. New York: McGraw-Hill Medical Pub. Division; 2014.

[3] Metellus, P; Barrie, M; Figarella-Branger, D; Chinot, O; Giorgi, R; Gouvernet, J; Jouvet, A; Guyotat, J. Multicentric French study on adult intracranial ependymomas: prognostic factors analysis and therapeutic considerations from a cohort of 152 patients. *Brain.* 2007 130, 1338-1349.

[4] Reni, M; Brandes, AA; Vavassori, V; Cavalo, G; Casagrande, F; Vastola, F et al. A multicenter study of the prognosis and treatment of adult brain ependymal tumors. *Cancer.* 2004 100, 1221-1229.

[5] Guyotat, J; Signorelli, F; Desme, S; et al. Intracranial ependymomas in adult patients: analyses or prognostic factors. *J. Neurooncol.* 2002 60(3), 255-268.

[6] Armstrong, TS; Vera-Bolanos, E; Bekele, BN; Aldape, K; Gilbert, MR. Adult ependymal tumors: prognosis and the M.D. Anderson Cencer Center experience. *Neuro-Oncology.* 2010 12(8), 862-870.

[7] Taylor, MD; Poppleton, H; Fuller, C; et al. Radial glia cells are candidate stem cells of ependymoma. *Cancer Cell* 2005 8, 323–335.

[8] Wani, K; Armstrong, TS; Vera-Bolanos, E; Raghunathan, A; Ellison, D; Gilbertson, R; Vaillant, B; Goldman, S; Packer, RJ; Fouladi, M; Pollack, I; Mikkelsen, T; Prados, M; Omuro, A; Soffietti, R; Ledoux, A; Wilson, C; Long, L;, Gilbert, MR; Aldape, K. A prognostic gene expression signature in infratentorial ependymoma. *Acta Neuropathologica.* 2010 123, 727-738.

[9] Benetto, L: Foreman, N; Harding, B; Hayward, R; Ironside, J; Love, S; Ellison, D. Ki-67 immunolabelling index is a prognostic indicator in childhood posterior fossa ependymomas. *Neuropathology and Applied Neurobiology.* 1998 24, 434-440.

[10] Altura, RA; Olshefski, RS; Jiang, Y; Boue, DR. Nuclear expression of Survivin in paediatric ependymomas and phoroid plexus tumours correlates with morphologic tumour grade. *British Journal of Cancer.* 2003 89, 1743-1749.

[11] Ridley, L; Rahman, R; Brundler, MA; Ellison, D; Lowe, J; Robson, K; Prebble, E; Luckett, I; Gilbertson, RJ; Parkes, S; Rand, V; Coyle, B; Grundy, RG. Multifactorial analysis of predictors of outcome in pediatric intracranial ependymoma. *Neuro-Oncol.* 2008 10(5), 675-689.

[12] Korshunov, A; Witt, K; Hielscher, T; Brenner, A; Remke, M; Ryzhova, M; Milde, T; Bender, S; Wittmann, A; Schottler, A; Kulozik, AE; von Deimling, A; Lichter, P; Pfister, S. Molecular staging of intracranial ependymoma in children and adults. *JCO.* 2010 28(19), 3182-3190.

[13] Pajtler, KW et al. Molecular classification of ependymal tumors across all CNS compartments, histopathological grades, and age groups. Cancer Cell 2015 27, 728-743.

[14] Archer, TC; Pomeroy, SL. Defining the molecular landscape of ependymomas. *Cancer Cell* 2015 27, 613-615.

[15] Parker, M; Mohankumar, KM; Punchihewa, C; Weinlich, R; Dalton, JD; Li, Y; Lee, R; Tatevossian, RG; Phoenix, TN; Thiruvenkatam, R; White, E; Tang, B; Orisme, W; Gupta, K; Rusch, M; Chen, X; Li, Y; Nagahawhatte, P; Hedlund, E; Finkelstein, D; Wu, G; Shurtleff, S; Easton, J; Boggs, K; Yergeau, D; et al. C11orf95-RELA fusions drive oncogenic NF-κB signaling in ependymoma. *Nature* 2014 506, 451-455.

[16] Gajjar, A; Pfister, SM; Taylor, MD; Gilbertson, RJ. Molecular insights into pediatric brain tumors have the potential to transform therapy. *Clin. Cancer Res.* 2014 20, 5630-5640.

[17] Mack, SC; Witt, H; Piro, RM; Gu, L; Zuyderduyn, S; Stutz, AM; Wang, X; Gallo, M; Garzia, L; Zayne, K; Zhang, X; Ramaswamy, V; Jager, N; Jones, DTW; Sill, M; Pugh, TJ; Ryzhova, M; Wani, KM; Shih, DJH; Head, R; Remke, M; Bailey, SD; Zichner, T; Faria, CC; Barszczyk, M, et al. Epigenomic alterations define lethal CIMP-positive ependymomas of infancy. *Nature* 2014 506, 445-450.

[18] Atkinson, JM; Shelatt, A; Carcaboso, AM; Kranenburg, TA; Arnold, LA; Boulos, N; et al. An integrated in vitro and in vivo high-throughput screen identifies leads for ependymoma. *Cancer Cell* 2011 20, 384-399.

[19] McGuire CS, Sainani KL, Fisher PG. Incidence patterns for ependymoma: a surveillance, epidemiology, and end results study. *J. Neurosurg.* 2009;110:725-729.

[20] Raghunathan, A; Wani, K; Armstrong, TS; Vera-Bolanos, E; Fouladi, M; Gilbertson, R; Gajjar, A; Goldman, S; Lehman, N; Metellus, P; Mikkelsen, T; Necesito-Reyes, MJT; Omuro, A; Packer, RJ; Partap, S; Pollack, IF; Prados, MD; Robins, HI; Soffietti, R; Wu, J; Miller, CRl Gilbert, MR; Aldape, KD. Histological predictors of outcome in ependymoma are dependent on anatomic site within the central nervous system. *Brain Pathology*. 2013 23, 584-594.

[21] Ernestus, RI; Schroder, R; Stutzer, H; Klug, N. The clinical and prognostic relevance of grading in intracranial ependymomas. *Br. J. Neurosurg.* 1997 11, 421-8.

[22] Oya, N; Shibamoto, Y; Nagata, Y; Negoro, Y; Hiraoka, M. Postoperative radiotherapy for intracranial ependymoma: analysis of prognostic factors and patterns of failure. *J. Neurooncol.* 2002 56, 87-94.

[23] Rogers, L; Pueschel, J; Spetzler, R; Shapiro, W; Coons, S; Thomas, T; et al. Is gross-total resection sufficient treatment for posterior fossa ependymomas? *J. Neurosurg.* 2005 102, 629-636.

[24] Iqbal, MS; Lewis, J. An overview of the management of adult ependymomas with emphasis on relapsed disease. *Clin. Oncol.* 2013 25(12), 726-733.

[25] Kawabata, Y; Takahashi, JA; Arakawa, Y; Hashimoto, N. Long-term outcome in patiets harboring intracranial ependymoma. *J. Neurosurg.* 2005 103(1), 31-37.

[26] Duffner, PK; Krischer, JP; Sanford, RA; Horowitz, ME; Burger, PC; Cohen, ME; Friedman, HS; Kun, LE. Prognostic factors in infants and very young children with intracranial ependymomas. *Pediatr Neurosurg.* 1998 28, 215-222.

[27] Reni, M; Gatta, G; Mazza, E; Vecht, C. Ependymoma. *Critical Reviews in Oncology/Hematology*. 2007 63, 81-89.

[28] Amirian, ES; Armstrong, TS; Gilbert, MR; Scheurer, ME. Predictors of survival among older adults with ependymoma. *J. Neurooncol.* 2012 107(1), 183-189.

[29] Chowdhary, S; Green, MR; Chamberlain, M. Ependymomas. *Curr. Treat Options Neurol.* 2006 8(4), 309-318.

[30] Bouffet, E; Hawkins, CE; Balloura, W. Survival benefit of pediatric patients with recurrent ependymoma treated with reirradiation. *Int. J. Radiat Oncol. Biol. Phys.* 2012 83(5), 1541-1548.

[31] Whitaker, SJ; Bessell, EM; Ashley, SE; Bloom, HJ; Bell, BA; Brada, M. Postoperative radiotherapy in the management of spinal cord ependymoma. *J. Neurosurg.* 1991 74, 720-728.

[32] Gomez, DR; Missett, BT; Wara, WM; Lamborn, KR; Prados, MD; Chang, S; Berger, MS; Haas-Kogan, DA. High failure rate in spinal ependymomas with long-term follow-up. *Neuro-Oncology*. 2005 7(3), 254-259.

In: Ependymomas
Editor: Raquel Fowler

ISBN: 978-1-63484-405-5

Chapter 2

PROGNOSTICATION, TREATMENT STRATEGIES AND CLINICAL OUTCOMES IN EPENDYMOMA DIAGNOSED PATIENTS

Damir Nizamutdinov[1,2], Kevin C. Graf[1], Samantha Dayawansa[1,2], Batool Kirmani[1,2], Erxi Wu[2], Jason H. Huang[1,2] and Ekokobe Fonkem[1,2]

[1]Texas A&M Health Science Center College of Medicine, Temple, TX, US
[2]Department of Neurosurgery, Baylor Scott and White Health, Temple, TX, US

ABSTRACT

Background and Purpose. Ependymoma is a rare primary brain tumor that arises from the ependymal cells of the intra-ventricular central nervous system (CNS) parenchyma with a propensity to affect both children and adults. This study aims to investigate the effects of gender, age, race, tumor grade, and treatment on clinical outcomes of ependymoma diagnosed patients.

Methods. Retrospective clinical analysis of ependymoma and systematic review of histological data were included in this study from the Scott and White Brain Tumor Registry collected from 1976-2013.

Results. About 30% of pediatric ependymomas were diagnosed in children younger than three years of age. Patients with completely resected tumors have an estimated 5-year survival rate of 67-80%, compared to an estimated 5-year survival rate of 22-47% in patients with incompletely resected tumors. Patients treated with post-operative radiation have a better outcome than patients who do not receive a radiation. Focal radiation to the site of the tumor lowers the risk of tumor recurrence at the site of origin. Ependymoma recurrence was observed in patients with grade III and II tumors. Ependymomas rarely metastasize outside of the CNS.

Most patients who deceased after treatment were under the age of 25. Pediatric 5-year survival rate was approximately 66% compared with the adult 5-year survival rate which was 78%. The 5-year male and female survival rates were in average of 80% and 60%, respectively. The 5-year survival rates of the White patients and patients of all other ethnicities as a single group were 73% and 75%, respectively. Patients with primary tumor sites in brain stem, frontal lobe, and parietal lobe have an excellent overall survival and low risk of tumor recurrence.

Conclusion. This study exhibits that surgical treatment with attempted gross total resection is a gold standard in treatment of ependymoma. The extent of surgical resection, age, and amount of tumor remaining after surgery are the primary factors influencing survival. Primary tumor site is another important prognostic factor for evaluation of short and long-term outcomes of ependymoma. Radiation therapy requires more future studies in order to elucidate more definitive treatment guidelines.

INTRODUCTION

Ependymoma is a primary brain tumor that arises from the ependymal cells of the intraventricular central nervous system (CNS) parenchyma. It is distinguishable from other CNS neoplasms by its rarity and its propensity to afflict children. (Vaidya, Smee, and Williams 2012) Histologically, ependymomas are moderately cellular gliomas with perivascular pseudo-rosettes, which is a term to describe tumor cells arranged radially around blood vessels with anuclear zones of fibrillary processes. Immunohistochemically, ependymomas express glial fibrillary acidic protein and display a characteristic dot-like cytoplasmic staining pattern with epithelial membrane antigen.

Ependymomas account for 6-10% of pediatric intracranial tumors and represent 2-6% of adult intracranial tumors (Massimino et al. 2006, Duffner et al. 1998, Rickert and Paulus 2001, Rodriguez et al. 2009, Villano, Parker, and Dolecek 2013, 2002). Among pediatric cohorts, supratentorial ependymomas are more common than infratentorial tumors and make up one third of all ependymomas, whereas infratentorial tumors are more common in adults (Rodriguez et al. 2009, Zacharoulis and Moreno 2009, Purdy et al. 2014, Amirian et al. 2012, McGuire, Sainani, and Fisher 2009). Currently, the 5-year survival rates from time of diagnosis for adults and children with ependymoma are 55-90% and 40-65%, respectively (Duffner et al. 1998, Rodriguez et al. 2009, Villano, Parker, and Dolecek 2013, Aizer et al. 2013, Horn et al. 1999). Several studies have analyzed survival rates of patients less than or equal to 3 years of age and these findings demonstrate that young children often have less favorable prognoses than adult or older pediatric patients (Purdy et al. 2014, Horn et al. 1999). This disparity can most likely be attributed to the fact that young children are often diagnosed when their disease has already progressed to a more advanced stage, thereby imparting a less favorable prognosis as compared to a patient whose ailment had been promptly observed and treated (Rickert and Paulus 2001). Few instances of extracranial metastasis have been recorded, but intraventricular metastases are relatively common with grade II and grade III tumor variants. In the World Health Organization (WHO) grading system, histopathological data classify ependymomas into 3 groups: grade I (subependymoma or myxopapillary ependymoma), grade II (classic ependymoma with cellular, papillary, clear cell, and tanycytic variants), and grade III (anaplastic) (Louis et al. 2007). Some ependymoma histopathological types are nearly always restricted in their areas of effect; an infratentorial subependymoma, for instance, has never been reported. Typically, ependymomas of the anaplastic variety are the most aggressive (Merchant et al. 1997, Phi et al. 2012). Some studies have concluded that prospective research should be continued on ependymomas before the anaplastic and classic varieties are more clearly delineated (Horn et al. 1999,

Merchant et al. 1997, Phi et al. 2012). However, patients presenting with subependymomas or classic ependymomas can still display bleak prognoses before treatment. With respect to subependymomas, the size and location of the tumor is most helpful in determining prognosis (Massimino et al. 2006, Duffner et al. 1998, Rickert and Paulus 2001, Rodriguez et al. 2009, McLaughlin et al. 1998, Rushing et al. 2007, Hou et al. 2013, Ragel et al. 2006, Scheithauer 1978). Symptoms of these tumors are generally the result of increased intracranial pressure due to obstructive hydrocephalus. The current gold standard of care for ependymoma treatment is gross total resection (GTR) with concurrent radiation therapy (RT), although studies have been done comparing the relative efficacy of GTR against subtotal resection (STR) in children and adults depending on the location of their ependymomas (infratentorial vs. supratentorial) (Merchant et al. 1997, Phi et al. 2012, McLaughlin et al. 1998, Rodriguez et al. 2009, Duffner et al. 1998, Aizer et al. 2013, Horn et al. 1999, Perilongo et al. 1997, Pollack et al. 1995). It has been shown that most recurrences following treatment are local, but RT decreases the probability of recurrence. The existence of relatively few ependymoma cases precludes the ability to reach any unassailable conclusions concerning appropriate treatment regimens, however most physicians agree that chemotherapy is relatively ineffective in enhancing progression-free survival (PFS) for ependymoma patients (Zacharoulis and Moreno 2009, Horn et al. 1999, Phi et al. 2012, Kim et al. 2004, Timmermann et al. 2000, Robertson et al. 1998, Evans et al. 1996).

This study aims to better understand prognostic value of different factors which can serve as reliable predictors of survival, treatment strategies, and clinical outcomes in ependymoma diagnosed patients. Findings are expected to add knowledge and change a current view on determination of outcomes in ependymoma patients.

Materials and Methods

Sources of Data and Study Population

All human investigations were performed after approval by an institutional review board and in accordance with an assurance filed with and approved by the U.S. Department of Health and Human Services.

Thirty-two clinical cases of ependymoma were obtained from the tumor registry of the Scott and White Integrated Healthcare System from 1976 to 2013. Age was categorized into two groups: children (less than or equal to 18 years) and adults (over 18). Race was categorized as white, Hispanic, black non-Hispanic, and other/unknown, with white vs. non-white also examined. Our categorization of tumor grade fell into 3 groups as determined by histopathological studies: grade I, grade II, and grade III. Data describing surgical method, RT, chemotherapy (CT), tumor recurrence, time to follow-up, were also included in data analysis. Surgical methods were described as STR, GTR, or no surgical procedure (NSP). RT and CT were described as either administered or not administered.

Data Analysis

The data were incorporated from an excel file into SAS, v9.2 (Cary, NC) and R, v2.15.1 (*The R Foundation for Statistical Computing*) to be analyzed for a number of variables. Descriptive statistics, including frequencies and percentages, were calculated to describe patient characteristics, tumor location, and mortality among ependymoma cases. Comparisons for mortality among locations were examined, overall and pairwise, using two-sample proportion tests. A type I error of $\alpha = 0.10$ was assumed throughout given the smaller size of 32 for the sample. Kaplan-Meier curves were drawn for overall statistics by gender, pediatric vs. adult, and white vs. other comparisons. Log-rank tests were used to compare mortality across groups. Quartile estimates of median survival time were carried out with difficulty due to the small sample sizes in use. Several of those median survival times lacked a lower or an upper 95% Confidence Interval as a result.

RESULTS

Twenty one (66%) patients were adults and the remaining eleven (34%) were under or equal to 18 years of age. Twenty-three patients (72%) were white, 5 (16%) Hispanic, 2 (6%) black and 2 (6%) other/unknown ethnicity. The majority of patients were male (59%). Three patients (9%) presented with grade III anaplastic ependymoma, 21 (66%) grade II ependymoma, and the remaining 8 (25%) had grade I subependymoma. Sixteen patients (50%) underwent STR, 11 (34%) GTR, and 5 (16%) underwent no surgical procedures. Among all 10 deceased patients, 8 (80%) underwent STR rather than GTR. Radiation therapy was administered in 50% of all cases, and chemotherapy in only 13%.

Eight patients (25% overall) became disease-free with no recurrence at the time of analysis. Two of them (25%) were treated only surgically. The remaining 6 (75%) were treated with a combination of surgery and radiation and/or chemotherapy. Among them, 5 were administered RT and 1 a combination of RT and CT. These efforts resulted in 5 being alive (63%) at a time of analysis. The remaining 3 deceased patients in this group underwent RT and were 2, 23 [2003], and 24 [2008] years of age at the (time of diagnosis), respectively. Among the 5 survivors, 2 were treated only surgically and were 18 [2001] and 24 [2012] years of age at the time of diagnosis, 2 underwent RT and were 1 [2003] and 46 [2010] years of age, and 1 patient underwent a combination of RT with CT and was 3 years of age in 2012 when first diagnosed. All 3 deceased patients were diagnosed with grade II tumors and the primary tumor sites were classified as, brain not otherwise specified (NOS) in 2 patients [2003, 2008] and brain stem in 1 patient [2003]. In comparison, 3 out of 5 living patients in this group were also diagnosed with grade II tumors and they were all treated surgically, but 2 also received RT. The primary tumor sites in these 3 patients were located in the frontal lobes in 2 [2001, 2003] and brain, NOS in 1 [2010]. One of the remaining 2 surviving individuals was diagnosed with a grade I tumor [2012] located in brain stem and underwent surgery alone, and another was diagnosed with grade III tumor [2012] located in parietal lobe and underwent surgery in combination with RT and CT.

Nine patients (28% overall) have never been disease-free after treatment. Seven surviving patients in this group received surgical treatments, among them 1 received additional RT, 2 were treated with RT and CT, and 4 underwent surgery alone. Two deceased patients (22%) underwent surgery and CT alone, respectively.

Tumor recurrence was reported in only 4 cases (13% overall), and all were grade II tumors, with 1 (25%) deceased. Data on tumor recurrence were unavailable for 11 patients. Among patients with unknown recurrence, 7 patients were diagnosed with grade II tumors, 3 with grade I tumors, and 1 with grade III tumor. Four (36%) were deceased by the time of data analysis.

Forty percent of deceased patients were under the age of 18. Our pediatric 5-year survival rate was 66% [95% Confidence Intervals (CI) 40-100%]. The adult 5-year survival rate was 78% (95% CI 58-100%). The median overall survival time for 32 reported cases was 15.2 years (182.5 months), and the 5-year survival rate was 80%. The median time to follow-up for those patients who are still living was 60.2 months, and the median time to follow-up for the deceased patients was 74.6 months.

Mortality by Tumor Location

We compared the incidence rates of the primary tumor sites between the total ependymoma diagnosed population, the subsistent treated, and deceased population to elucidate possible survival trends. A side-by-side comparison is shown in Figure 1. These data suggest a survival rate of 88% observed with primary tumor sites located in the brain stem versus 63% elsewhere (p = 0.186; Table 1). Survival with tumors located in the frontal lobe was 100% versus 66% in other locations (p = 0.220), and with 100% survival for parietal lobe (p = 0.325).

Table 1. Mortality rate overall and by location. Overall average for survivors was 69% of the sample. Among survivors, brain stem (32%) and ventricle, NOS (23.0%) were most prevalent locations. Overall average for deceased patients was 31%. Among the deceased, mortality was greater for brain, NOS (57%), temporal lobe (50%), and ventricle, NOS (38%). Cerebrum location (1 case) resulted in death. Lower rates of mortality were observed for the brain stem, frontal lobe, and parietal lobe with a single case for cerebellum surviving. A significant difference in mortality was observed for brain, NOS versus other locations (57% vs. 24%, p = 0.094)

Location	Total (N = 32) N (%)	Alive (N = 22, 68.8%) N (%)	Dead (N = 10, 31.3%) N (%)	Mortality Rate %	P-value
Brain stem	8 (25.0)	7 (31.8)	1 (10.0)	12.5	0.186
Brain, NOS	7 (21.9)	3 (13.6)	4 (40.0)	57.1	0.094
Cerebellum, NOS	1 (3.1)	1 (4.5)	0 (0.0)	0.0	0.493
Cerebrum	1 (3.1)	0 (0.0)	1 (10.0)	100	0.132
Frontal lobe	3 (9.4)	3 (13.6)	0 (0.0)	0.0	0.220
Parietal lobe	2 (6.3)	2 (9.1)	0 (0.0)	0.0	0.325
Temporal lobe	2 (6.3)	1 (4.5)	1 (10.0)	50.0	0.555
Ventricle, NOS	8 (25.0)	5 (22.7)	3 (30.0)	37.5	0.660

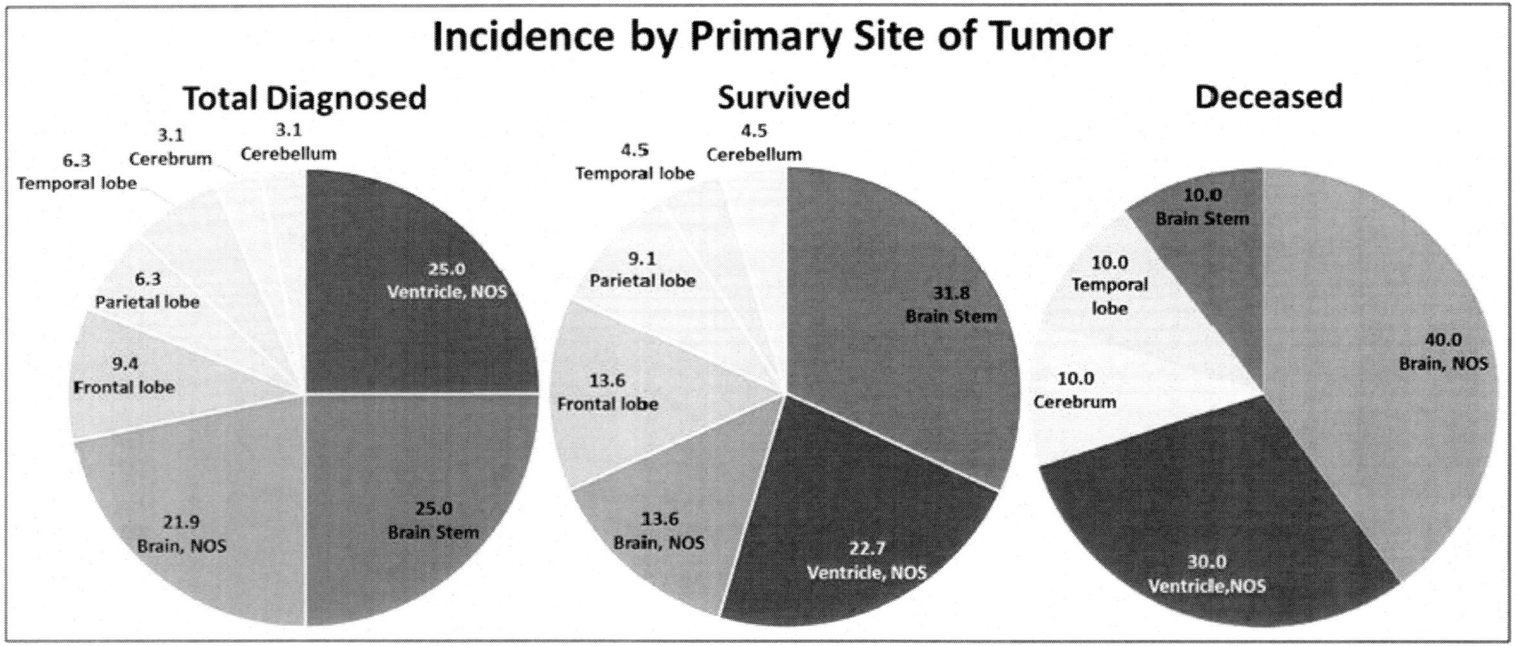

Figure 1. Comparative analysis of primary tumor sites in ependymoma total diagnosed patients vs. survived vs. deceased patients at the time of data analysis. Total number of 32 cases were analyzed using R, ver. 2.15.1. Ependymoma was located in the ventricle NOS (25% vs. 23%, p = 0.660), in brain stem (25% vs. 32%, p = 0.186), in brain, NOS (22% vs. 14%, p = 0.094), in frontal lobe (9% vs.14%, p = 0.220), in parietal lobe (6% vs. 9%, p = 0.325), in temporal lobe (6% vs. 5%, p = 0.555), in cerebrum (3% vs. 0%, p = 0.132), and in cerebellum (3% vs. 5%, p = 0.493), respectively.

Table 2. Pairwise comparisons of mortality rates among locations. Test represents significantly lower mortality rate for brain stem compared to brain, NOS (13% vs. 57%, p = 0.067), to cerebrum (13% vs. 100%, p = 0.047), respectively. Greater mortality of brain, NOS was significant compared to locations in frontal lobe (57% vs. 0%, p = 0.091). Cerebrum showed significantly greater rates of mortality compared to frontal lobe (100% vs. 0%, p = 0.046) and to temporal lobe (100% vs. 0%, p = 0.083), respectively

Pairwise P-values	**Brain stem** n = 8	**Brain NOS** n = 7	**Cerebellum NOS** n = 1	**Cere-brum** n = 1	**Frontal lobe** n = 3	**Parietal lobe** n = 2	**Temporal lobe** n = 2	**Ventricle NOS** n = 8
Mortality:	**12.5%**	**57.1%**	**0.0%**	**100%**	**0.0%**	**0.0%**	**50.0%**	**37.5%**
Location n, Mortality								
Brain stem n = 8, **12.5%**	---	0.067	0.708	0.047	0.521	0.598	0.236	0.248
Brain, NOS n = 7, **57.1%**		---	0.285	0.408	0.091	0.151	0.858	0.447
Cerebellum, NOS n = 1, **0.0%**			---	0.157	NA	NA	0.386	0.453
Cerebrum n = 1, **100%**				---	0.046	0.083	0.386	0.236
Frontal lobe n = 3, **0.0%**					---	NA	0.171	0.214
Parietal lobe n = 2, **0.0%**						---	0.248	0.301
Temporal lobe n = 2, **50.0%**							---	0.747
Ventricle, NOS n = 8, **37.5%**								---

Among patients who died, accounting for 31% of all cases (Table 1), the most prevalent location was brain, NOS (40%), followed by ventricle, NOS (30%). Among survivors, accounting for the remaining 69% of the sample, brain stem (32%) and ventricle, NOS (23%) were most prevalent locations. Mortality was greater for brain, NOS (57%), temporal lobe (50%), and ventricle, NOS (38%) compared to the overall average of 31%. There was one case involving the cerebrum, which resulted in death. Lower rates were observed for the brain stem, frontal lobe, and parietal lobe with a single case for cerebellum surviving. A significant difference in mortality was observed for brain, NOS versus other locations (57% vs. 24%, p = 0.094).

Pairwise comparisons among tumor locations (Table 2) revealed a significantly lower mortality rate for brain stem compared to brain, NOS (13% vs. 57%, p = 0.067), and compared to cerebrum (13% vs. 100%, p = 0.047). Brain, NOS also resulted in greater mortality than frontal lobe (57% vs. 0%, p = 0.091). Cerebrum had higher rates of mortality versus both frontal and parietal lobe (100% vs. 0% for both, p = 0.046 and p = 0.083), respectively.

Conclusion

Physicians are currently trying to discern the most effective treatments for ependymoma patients. Due to the rarity of its occurrence, researchers must rely on a paucity of information that can only be retrospectively analyzed. Our results still offer plenty of talking points from the standpoint of a systematic review.

Considering surgical excision with attempted GTR is the current gold standard for ependymoma treatment, the administration of concurrent RT is contingent upon the extent of resection, tumor grade, patient age, and the presence or absence of tumor dissemination, which would most commonly occur through the cerebrospinal fluid (Aizer et al. 2013, Korshunov et al. 2004, Rogers et al. 2005, Merchant et al. 2009, Mansur et al. 2005, English 2009, Awaad et al. 1996).

Some studies have demonstrated that STR is more effective in treatment of infratentorial and adult ependymomas. From the first of these criteria, we can infer that the tumor location relates to the size of the infratentorial space as compared to the supratentorial space. STR excises less tissue and is therefore less likely to cause comorbidities. Considering the latter of the two criteria, loss of brain tissue from an adult confers greater risk than it would be for a comparable loss in a child due to neuroplasticity concerns. Despite these findings, it is generally accepted that GTR is more effective in fully eradicating the disease regardless of the patient's age and tumor location.

The deceased patient group had a longer median time to follow up than the patients who are still alive. We expected to see this kind of relationship since cancer becomes steadily more difficult to treat the longer it goes unmonitored.

Even though our survival rates were consistent with the current standards, our confidence intervals were wide, meaning that our survival estimates were not very precise. This can be attributed to the small sample size.

Recurrence data were not reported for 11 patients, but it is not unusual for patients whose symptoms have dissipated to neglect contact with the healthcare system. Recurrence was seen in only 4 of the patients (13%), but could very well have been present in any of the 7 patients with grade II tumors and/or 1 patient with grade III tumor whose recurrence statuses were unknown. Recurrence was seen in all 4 of the ependymoma, NOS cases.

Cranial variants of ependymoma have a less favorable outcome than primary spinal cord ependymomas (McGuire, Sainani, and Fisher 2009). Location within the spinal cord may also affect outcome, with tumors in the lower portion of the spinal cord having a worse prognosis (Safaee et al. 2014).

Among 8 patients who became disease-free with no recurrence after treatment, 3 deceased. All three underwent combination of surgery and RT treatment and were diagnosed with grade II tumor with primary tumor sites located in the brain stem (1 patient) and brain, NOS (2 patients). Among the 5 living individuals in this group, 2 were diagnosed with grade II tumors and underwent a combination of surgery and RT treatment. Both were the same age and had the same time of first diagnosis, compared with deceased patients in this group. Although the age, diagnosis, time of diagnosis, and treatment between deceased and alive individuals were all the same, the primary tumor sites between these 2 groups were different. In living individuals, the primary tumor sites were in the frontal lobes (2 patients) and the brain, NOS (1 patient).

When the data for a total diagnosed ependymoma population was analyzed based on tumor primary site and compared with living patients who underwent treatment, it was found that treatment of ependymoma located in the brain stem, frontal lobe, and parietal lobe had significantly greater survival and recurrence-free outcomes than tumors located in the brain, NOS, cerebrum or ventricle, NOS.

Since 80% of the patients who died underwent STR rather than GTR, GTR could perhaps have been attempted on some of those patients. However, we do not know whether the cases in which patients underwent STR instead of GTR were intentional or accidental. Additionally, we know that a partial resection is defined as removal of 1 or less lobes of a tumor. As such, some of our data labeled as STR may have in fact been GTR depending on the nature of the tumor architecture, ignoring that GTR is not in itself a guarantee of absolute resection. For the purposes of this study, partial resections were taken to be STR despite the possibility of error. STR is sometimes a better choice than GTR if the physician wishes to decrease the risk of debilitating morbidity to the patient (Zacharoulis and Moreno 2009, Safaee et al. 2014, Ideguchi et al. 2013, Li et al. 2014). On the other hand, such a treatment choice can lower the survival time of the patient. This dichotomy exists for many cancer therapy choices, and healthcare professionals are still searching for new treatment options that both promote longevity and provide palliative relief.

Seventy percent of deceased patients were under the age of 25, which could perhaps suggest a more appropriate cut-off than those currently in use (less than or equal to 21 years and over 21). However, stratification by age can prove difficult. Most would consider pediatric groups to encompass those 18 years of age or younger, but some groups - the American Cancer Society, for instance - take the pediatric qualifier to be 19 years or younger (2014). Research has shown that the onset of neuroplasticity can occur in the late 20's, which may be of some concern to those conducting future studies that compare child to adult.

We know that recurrence is relatively common in with grade III ependymoma, and it is not uncommon with grade II tumors. So our grade I patients whose recurrence statuses were unknown are not necessarily important to this study. Subependymomas are generally well-circumscribed and well-differentiated, thus surgical resection with or without concurrent radiotherapy is usually very effective in conferring a good long-term prognosis (Rushing et al. 2007). Anaplastic ependymomas are considered to be the most likely to metastasize, recur, and to diminish overall survival (OS). If we had a greater breadth of anaplastic patients, or data may have yielded differential results. Studies show anywhere from 42% to 100% recurrence in grade III ependymoma (Merchant et al. 2002, Roldan Urgoiti et al. 2014, Massimino et al. 2004, Oya et al. 2002). Four additional cases of recurrence occurred among patients with grade II ependymoma, which is less common than it is for grade III, but not so uncommon as to be surprising. In 50% of the cases, RT was administered, but in only 13% of the cases was chemotherapy administered. This corresponds with the current standard of ependymoma treatment. Chemotherapy has not been found to decrease instance of tumor recurrence with ependymoma or to enhance the patient's PFS; rather, studies have shown that occasionally it can even exacerbate progression of the tumor by conferring natural selection and thereby resistant qualities upon the tumor cells (Bergers and Hanahan 2008, Fischer et al. 2013). RT administration was also found to be consistent with expectations. Each of the 3 anaplastic cases was given radiotherapy, 13 of 21 (62%) grade II cases had radiotherapy administered, and none of the subependymoma cases underwent any kind of radiotherapy. Anaplastic ependymoma is the most likely to metastasize and/or recur of the three tumor grades, and so it was necessary to irradiate the brain tissue in all of those cases. Grade II ependymomas can fall anywhere on a wide spectrum from benign to aggressive brain tumors, so it was not surprising to see a large split in that group of patients regarding RT administration. It would have been nonsensical to administer radiotherapy on the patients presenting with subependymoma, and indeed we see that none of those patients were irradiated. Despite the consistency between our findings and other studies, no correlation was found to exist between mortality and the administration of radiotherapy. Seven of the grade II patients who were given radiotherapy are deceased, while the remaining 9 who received radiotherapy (6 of the grade II and the 3 of the grade III patients) are alive. Thirteen of the patients who did not receive radiotherapy are still alive, although it should be noted that 8 of those patients presented with subependymoma. Our analysis showed that 66% of the patients had grade II tumors.

We would likely have utilized an additional age cut-off of 25 but for statistical deficits due to the fact that neurological development has been tracked well past 18 years of age. Our results still conform to the current standards for 5-year survival rates, but if we had been able to derive any statistical significance from the aforementioned age cut-off, we may have in fact discovered a more precise correlation between age and survival rate. We could also render more precision unto the study by having similar group sizes for adults and children. In fact, older ependymoma studies demonstrate some of the issues that can accompany preference of one group over the other. Ependymoma research used to consist almost solely of pediatric studies (Kilday et al. 2009, Mack and Taylor 2009). Although adult cases are generally less serious, a large group of clinical cases for an erratic and unpredictable diseases were not seriously considered for study. By maintaining a close ratio in children to adults for future ependymoma studies, we believe that results will be more indicative of pathological factors than they would be with a resolute focus on one age group or the other.

Ependymoma can be quite injurious to a patient's health, or it can reside in the intraventricular spaces for many years without causing serious health risks. In either case, recurrent disease after treatment often carries a poor prognosis, regardless of the tendency of recurrence to be local. However, radiation administered in the form of focal irradiation, stereotactic radiosurgery, or craniospinal radiotherapy has led to the current 5-year survival rates of both children and adults, which are greatly increased from earlier records (32% in 1986, 51% in 1990, and 64% in 1998) (Rickert and Paulus 2001, Preston-Martin 1996, Bloom et al. 1990).

Fortunately, these survival rates are higher than those of many other CNS cancers, as we will soon show. The median overall survival time of our patients was 15.2 years (182.51 months), and our survival curve estimates an 80% 5 year survival rate for our 32 patients. According to the American Cancer Society (ACS), ependymoma has a greater 5-year survival rate in all adult age groups than the other common brain tumor types, with the exception of meningioma in the 20-44 age group, which has a 5-year survival rate of 92%. The values for ependymoma as delineated by the ACS are 91% for patients ages 20-44, 86% for 45-54, and 85% for 55-64. The ACS has also published pediatric 5-year survival rates that demonstrate ependymoma has the 4th worst rate among child brain tumors with a value of 75% (the pediatric qualifier here taken to be those patients aged 19 years and younger) (2014). Thus, while ependymoma is generally accepted to be one of the less serious types of brain cancer, it can often carry quite unfavorable prognoses in children. Our study demonstrates a lower pediatric 5-year survival rate of 66% in children, while the adult group showed a 5-year survival rate of 78%, which is slightly lower than might be expected upon examination of the rates released by the American Cancer Society. However, our results correlate with the widely accepted 5-year survival rate intervals that are cited by many ependymoma studies, which are 55-90% for adults and 40-65% for children. Our values of 78% and 66%, respectively, may illustrate the recent progress that has been made in cancer treatments. Time to surgery and time to radiation numbers would have been helpful determinants of survival rate relationships as well, but reporting standards unfortunately did not necessitate the recording of these values for enough of our patients. However, as previously discussed, we can see a clear relationship between time to follow up and mortality. The median time to follow up was 60.24 months for those patients still living and 74.58 months for those deceased.

Upfront RT was also found to increase OS and it is suggested that more aggressive treatments should almost always be pursued in the case of adult ependymoma, which indicates a possible advantage of upfront RT after maximal surgical resection. This concurs with previous results by the Pediatric Oncology Group (POG) "Baby POG" study that examined 48 children less than the age of 3 years with intracranial ependymoma treated with prolonged post-operative chemotherapy and delayed RT. Their study suggests that OS was significantly worse in the younger group (P ¼ 0.04), with a 5-year OS of only 26% in patients less than 2 years when compared with 63% in those between 2 and 3 years.

Despite recent results indicating relative safety of irradiation during young childhood with regard to neurocognitive performance (Amirian et al. 2012, Merchant et al. 1997), one should be vigilant about the short and long term adverse effects of irradiation. The use of conformal RT in 87 pediatric patients with ependymoma was associated with a small but significant decline in word reading scores but not spelling and math reasoning, with age at RT less than 5 years being predictive of such decline (Robertson et al. 1998). Acquired attention deficit was also apparent in a pediatric and young adult cohort with brain tumor after conformal RT (Evans et al. 1996). In light of such research and findings, radiation is typically excluded from treatments for children less than 3 years old. Continued follow-up of this vulnerable patient group is essential for the surveillance of longer-term neurocognitive impairment and other deleterious effects on growth, puberty, endocrine functions, hearing loss, and secondary malignancies. The use of re-irradiation in relapse treatment poses additional risk for short and long-term adverse effects, in particular radiation necrosis for those undergoing hypofractionated RT or stereotactic radiosurgery (Timmermann et al. 2000, Rogers et al. 2005).

Anaplastic ependymomas are considered to be a greater threat concerning intraventricular metastasis, but very few studies have been able to corroborate this statement, and our 3 patients with anaplastic ependymomas are interestingly still alive. Ependymomas are elegantly unpredictable in this manner. The anaplastic patients in our study may represent a special scenario for treatment considering the following three regimens as recorded in our data: 1) no surgical procedure, no chemotherapy administered, RT administered; 2) GTR, chemotherapy administered, RT administered; 3) no surgical procedure, chemotherapy administered, RT administered. Each of the 3 cases saw a distinctive treatment regime. The first of these cases could not have employed chemotherapy since the diagnosis and primary treatment occurred in 1985, but the variety in treatment still presents an interesting idea. In each of these cases there was no recurrence, which could demonstrate that location and age contribute to prognosis more so than do histopathological qualities of the tumor. Studies still disagree on the differences that separate classic ependymomas from those of the anaplastic variety (many physicians rely on consensus histopathology). Having said that, we also recognize that tumor grade is statistically significant in our study. Yet, only patients with grade II tumors experienced mortality. Future studies should place emphasis on ependymomas of the anaplastic variety. Less surprising was the finding that patients diagnosed with subependymomas did not experience mortality. Survival rates for subependymoma are generally higher than those of grade II or grade III (Amirian et al. 2012, Merchant et al. 2002, Roldan Urgoiti et al. 2014). Neither the 8 patients with subependymoma nor the 3 patients with anaplastic tumors have died, and we already know that we cannot attribute the survival of those 3 anaplastic cases to a single treatment regimen. Random effects of other variables may have prevented the deaths of the 3 anaplastic patients, but it is unlikely that all 8 subependymoma patients have survived since diagnosis due to chance. So we conclude that tumor grade can be an important prognostic consideration when comparing grade I to grade II tumors, but our data yielded little else to derive other conclusions therein.

Some studies have shown that chemotherapy can delay progression and provide palliative relief to patients with ependymoma, but it has not been found to increase survival (Timmermann et al. 2000, Robertson et al. 1998, Evans et al. 1996, Massimino et al. 2004). Ependymomas express vascular endothelial growth factor (VEGF), and certain chemotherapies inhibit this growth factor to delay progression of the tumor in question. However, in cases of anti-angiogenesis therapies, resistance may be conferred to daughter cells of those cells that survived the therapy. One study has even proffered the idea that chemotherapy may promote metastases on a long-term basis (Bergers and Hanahan 2008). The point here is that up-regulation of alternative pathways of angiogenesis may compensate for and nullify the initial positive effects of chemotherapy such that survival rates remain constant and consistent.

cDNA-based microarrays have been used to assess gene expression in ependymomas. The most frequent DNA copy number variants in ependymomas include a gain of chromosome 1 or a loss of chromosome 22, but there is a high degree of heterogeneity in gene expression among ependymoma cases (Kilday et al. 2009, Mack and Taylor 2009, Mazewski et al. 1999). One study identified 56 differentially expressed genes and compared their proliferation indices to survival rate, patient age, histopathology, and tumor location. Correlations were found only between subtypes of grade I tumors (subependymomas and myxopapillary ependymomas) and in the survival rate of children. No correlation was discovered between gene expression and tumor grade (grade I vs. grade II vs. grade III) or patient age at diagnosis (Lukashova-V. Zangen et al. 2007).

Some case reports indicate the pathogenesis of extraventicular ependymomas, but the results of these publications do not promote any general conclusions. We do know, however, that myxopapillary ependymoma only manifests itself in the spine. It has been seen in no other area of the CNS (Nakamura et al. 2009, Shirasawa et al. 2014).

Age associated observation in our study shows that 66% of the patients were adults and only 34% were children. These numbers do not agree with the theme that ependymoma is more commonly seen in children. These numbers also made it impossible to find a correlation between any of our given variables and the pediatric cohort, which would have allowed a comparison to the effect of that variable on the adult cohort.

Thus far, the influence of gender has not been thoroughly investigated in ependymoma studies because it almost equally afflicts men and women and progresses similarly in both.

Our study showed an 80% 5-year survival rate for males and a 60% for females, but these values are probably trivial. A larger study would most likely demonstrate more similar 5-year survival rates among males and females.

Another neglected survival relationship is ependymoma outcome by race. Our results show that there was no statistical significance in the white vs. non-white analysis. Our study showed that the 5-year survival rate was 73% for white patients and 75% for the other races as one single grouping. Despite the similarity in mortality between these groups, a correlation may exist between ethnicity and ependymoma development since 72% of our 32 patients were white. However, we know that all of the patients in our study are from Central Texas, and, considering the demographics of that region, there could very well be a genetic correlation between ependymoma development and white ethnicity, although no genetic markers of this sort have been discovered as of yet. To expound, whites are less predominant in Central Texas than are Hispanics, and so the fact that we saw more whites afflicted than any other race possibly denotes a genetic indicator. Going forward, it would be helpful to survey ependymoma cases in several distinct regions, each dominated by a specific demographic so as to garner a more valuable statistical perspective.

It would be helpful to raise larger cohorts for continued study of ependymomas. Healthcare data aggregation is paramount to successful prospective studies, as is strict adherence to pre-designated reporting standards. Reports concerning intracranial tumor resection and adjuvant RT should be especially definitive. One specific example of these difficulties is the very recent development of pseudo-universal computerization; large-scale movements of charting systems have thereby muddled our ability to assert the specific differences between certain treatment regimens. Some of these reforms have dictated that reporting standards be changed so that the definition of surgery methods, for instance, present contradictory or overlapping information. So movements to regulate these areas would aid in the delegation of more significant retrospective studies. The reporting standards have changed since the 1970s, for instance, and so it can be difficult to assert the difference between local excision and STR.

What we glean more assuredly from this study is that there seems to be a higher incidence of ependymoma among white populations. And, considering the demographics of Central Texas, there could very well be a genetic correlation between white ethnicity and ependymoma development, although prospective studies need to be pursued in order to confirm this hypothesis. As far as finding a standard of care, our study shows that resection with concurrent RT is an effective tool in conferring PFS, but chemotherapy is negligibly effectual, most likely due to movement inhibitions incited by the blood brain barrier. Despite the fact that some physicians continue to use chemotherapy for ependymoma cases, this study asserts the trend that resection with adjuvant radiation is the best standard. The deficit in ependymoma cases and studies makes it difficult to conclude anything more definitive, but our study suggest that tumor grade is more important than age or location of the tumor in a physician's consideration of how to treat ependymoma cases, but only concerning grade II and grade III tumors. Subependymoma cases are usually going to carry very different prognoses that are concerned more with age and location (Rushing et al. 2007, Hou et al. 2013, Ragel et al. 2006, Scheithauer 1978). Since tumor grade may be subject to change in the future, age and location of the tumor are likely to be more important prognostic indicators in current consideration. Had this study been conducted with more statistical power, we perhaps would have seen different results. It remains true, however, that ependymomas are difficult to predict. In light of these facts, and because our patients' treatment regimens seldom included chemotherapy, we only considered surgery and RT in their respective and collective capacities to halt the progression of or fully eradicate ependymomas in our patients. There does seem to be a correlation between mortality and surgery type in that gross total resection confers better prognosis and PFS as opposed to subtotal resection, but administration of RT does not seem to relate to survival, at least in the capacity that it normally serves within the healthcare system. What this means is that the only patients who died and also did not receive radiotherapy (with the exception of one 59 year old woman) were less than 3 years old. Radiation is very seldom given to children less than 3 years old because it is considered to be too neurodegenerative.

There has been little discussion concerning the merits of time to surgery or time to radiation. More information on these factors would be helpful for future studies. Moving forward, ependymoma should be treated with a careful eye for unusual circumstances, as any resulting case studies could lend more credence to ongoing prospective studies.

In conclusion, one of the major factors which affect overall survival and can be used as a reliable prognostic tool in groups of patients diagnosed with ependymoma is a location of primary tumor. Surgical treatment with attempted gross total resection is a gold standard in treatment of ependymoma. The primary tumor sites in brain stem, frontal lobe, and parietal lobe seem to have an excellent outcome in terms of survival and recurrence of disease when treated surgically. There seems to be a genetic correlation between ependymoma development and white ethnicity.

Acknowledgments

This study was supported by NIH grant: R01-NS067435.

References

2002. *Primary brain tumors in the United States: statistical report*, 1995-1999. CBTRUS.

2014. *Cancer in children and adolescents*. Atlanta: American Cancer Society.

Aizer, A. A., Ancukiewicz M., Nguyen P. L., Macdonald S. M., Yock T. I., Tarbell N. J., Shih H. A., Loeffler J. S. and Oh K. S., 2013. Natural history and role of radiation in patients with supratentorial and infratentorial WHO grade II ependymomas: results from a population-based study. *J Neurooncol* 115 (3):411-9. doi:10.1007/s11060-013-123 7-9.

Amirian, E. S., Armstrong T. S., Aldape K. D., Gilbert M. R., and Scheurer M. E., 2012. Predictors of survival among pediatric and adult ependymoma cases: a study using Surveillance, Epidemiology, and End Results data from 1973 to 2007. *Neuroepidemiology* 39 (2):116-24. doi:10.1159/0003 39320.

Awaad, Y. M., Allen J. C., Miller D. C., Schneider S. J., Wisoff J., and Epstein F. J., 1996. Deferring adjuvant therapy for totally resected intracranial ependymoma. *Pediatr Neurol* 14 (3):216-19.

Bergers, G., and Hanahan D., 2008. Modes of resistance to anti-angiogenic therapy. *Nat Rev Cancer* 8 (8):592-603. doi: 10.1038/nrc2442.

Bloom, H. J., Glees J., Bell J., Ashley S. E., and Gorman C., 1990. The treatment and long-term prognosis of children with intracranial tumors: a study of 610 cases, 1950-1981. *Int J Radiat Oncol Biol Phys* 18 (4):723-45.

Duffner, P. K., Krischer J. P., Sanford R. A., Horowitz M. E., Burger P. C., Cohen M. E., Friedman H. S., and Kun L. E., 1998. Prognostic factors in infants and very young children with intracranial ependymomas. *Pediatr Neurosurg* 28 (4):215-22.

English, M. W. 2009. 21st century management of ependymoma. *Lancet Oncol* 10 (3):206-7. doi:10.1016/S1470-2045(09)70052-X.

Evans, A. E., Anderson J. R., Lefkowitz-Boudreaux I. B., and Finlay J. L., 1996. Adjuvant chemotherapy of childhood posterior fossa ependymoma: cranio-spinal irradiation with or without adjuvant CCNU, vincristine, and prednisone: a Childrens Cancer Group study. *Med Pediatr Oncol* 27 (1):8-14. doi:10.1002/(SICI)1096-911X(199607)27:1<8::AID-MPO3>3.0.CO; 2-K.

Fischer, C., Haque S. S., Huse J. T., Blochin E., Souweidane M. M., Lis E., and Khakoo Y., 2013. Extraneural ependymoma: distant bone, lung, liver, and lymph node metastases following bevacizumab. *Pediatr Blood Cancer* 60 (1):143-5. doi:10.1002/pbc.24268.

Horn, B., Heideman R., Geyer R., Pollack I., Packer R., Goldwein J., Tomita T., Schomberg P., Ater J., Luchtman-Jones L., Rivlin K., Lamborn K., Prados M., Bollen A., Berger M., Dahl G., McNeil E., Patterson K., Shaw D., Kubalik M., and Russo C., 1999. A multi-institutional retrospective study of intracranial ependymoma in children: identification of risk factors. *J Pediatr Hematol Oncol* 21 (3):203-11.

Hou, Z., Z. Wu, J. Zhang, L. Zhang, R. Tian, B. Liu, and Z. Wang. 2013. Clinical features and management of intracranial subependymomas in children. *J Clin Neurosci* 20 (1):84-8. doi:10.1016/j.jocn.2012.05.026.

Ideguchi, M., Kajiwara K., Yoshikawa K., Sadahiro H., Nomura S., Fujii M., and Suzuki M., 2013. Characteristics of intraoperative abnormal hemodynamics during resection of an intra-fourth ventricular tumor located on the dorsal medulla oblongata. *Neurol Med Chir* (Tokyo) 53 (10):655-62.

Kilday, J. P., Rahman R., Dyer S., Ridley L., Lowe J., Coyle B., and Grundy R., 2009. Pediatric ependymoma: biological perspectives. *Mol Cancer Res* 7 (6):765-86. doi:10.1158/1541-7786.MCR-08-0584.

Kim, S. K., Lim S. Y., Wang K. C., Kim Y. Y., Chi J. G., Choi Y. L., Shin H. J., and Cho B. K., 2004. Overexpression of cyclooxygenase-2 in childhood ependymomas: role of COX-2 inhibitor in growth and multi-drug resistance *in vitro*. *Oncol Rep* 12 (2):403-9.

Korshunov, A., Golanov A., Sycheva R., and Timirgaz V., 2004. The histologic grade is a main prognostic factor for patients with intracranial ependymomas treated in the microneurosurgical era: an analysis of 258 patients. *Cancer* 100 (6):1230-7. doi:10.1002/cncr.20075.

Li, T. Y., Chu J. S., Xu Y. L., Yang J., Wang J., Huang Y. H., Kwan A. L., and Wang G. H., 2014. Surgical strategies and outcomes of spinal ependymomas of different lengths: analysis of 210 patients: clinical article. *J Neurosurg Spine* 21 (2):249-59. doi:10.3171/2014.3.SPINE134 81.

Louis, D. N., Ohgaki H., Wiestler O. D., Cavenee W. K., Burger P. C., Jouvet A., Scheithauer B. W., and Kleihues P., 2007. The 2007 WHO classification of tumours of the central nervous system. *Acta Neuropathol* 114 (2):97-109. doi:10.1007/s00401-007-0243-4.

Lukashova-V. Zangen, I., Kneitz S., Monoranu C. M., Rutkowski S., Hinkes B., Vince G. H., Huang B., and Roggendorf W., 2007. Ependymoma gene expression profiles associated with histological subtype, proliferation, and patient survival. *Acta Neuropathol* 113 (3):325-37. doi:10.1007/s00401-006-0190-5.

Mack, S. C., and Taylor M. D., 2009. The genetic and epigenetic basis of ependymoma. *Childs Nerv Syst* 25 (10):1195-201. doi:10.1007/s00381-009-0928-1.

Mansur, D. B., Perry A., Rajaram V., Michalski J. M., Park T. S., Leonard J. R., Luchtman-Jones L., Rich K. M., Grigsby P. W., Lockett M. A., Wahab S. H., and Simpson J. R., 2005. Postoperative radiation therapy for grade II and III intracranial ependymoma. *Int J Radiat Oncol Biol Phys* 61 (2): 387-91. doi: 10.1016/j.ijrobp.2004.06.002.

Massimino, M., Gandola L., Giangaspero F., Sandri A., Valagussa P., Perilongo G., Garre M. L., Ricardi U., Forni M., Genitori L., Scarzello G., Spreafico F., Barra S., Mascarin M., Pollo B., Gardiman M., Cama A., Navarria P., Brisigotti M., Collini P., Balter R., Fidani P., Stefanelli M., Burnelli R., Potepan P., Podda M., Sotti G., Madon E., and Aieop Pediatric Neuro-Oncology Group. 2004. Hyperfractionated radiotherapy and chemotherapy for childhood ependymoma: final results of the first prospective AIEOP (Associazione Italiana di Ematologia-Oncologia Pediatrica) study. *Int J Radiat Oncol Biol Phys* 58 (5):1336-45. doi:10. 1016/j.ijrobp.2003.08.030.

Massimino, M., Giangaspero F., Garre M. L., Genitori L., Perilongo G., Collini P., Riva D., Valentini L., Scarzello G., Poggi G., Spreafico F., Peretta P., Mascarin M., Modena P., Sozzi G., Bedini N., Biassoni V., Urgesi A., Balestrini M. R., Finocchiaro G., Sandri A., Gandola L., and Aieop Neuro-Oncology Group. 2006. Salvage treatment for childhood ependymoma after surgery only: Pitfalls of omitting 'at once' adjuvant treatment. *Int J Radiat Oncol Biol Phys* 65 (5):1440-5. doi:10.1016/j. ijrobp.2006.03.052.

Mazewski, C., Soukup S., Ballard E., Gotwals B., and Lampkin B., 1999. Karyotype studies in 18 ependymomas with literature review of 107 cases. *Cancer Genet Cytogenet* 113 (1):1-8.

McGuire, C. S., Sainani K. L., and Fisher P. G., 2009. Incidence patterns for ependymoma: a surveillance, epidemiology, and end results study. *J Neurosurg* 110 (4):725-9. doi:10.3171/2008.9.JNS08117.

McLaughlin, M. P., Marcus R. B., Jr., Buatti J. M., McCollough W. M., Mickle J. P., Kedar A., Maria B. L., and Million R. R., 1998. Ependymoma: results, prognostic factors and treatment recommendations. *Int J Radiat Oncol Biol Phys* 40 (4):845-50.

Merchant, T. E., Haida T., Wang M. H., Finlay J. L., and Leibel S. A., 1997. Anaplastic ependymoma: treatment of pediatric patients with or without craniospinal radiation therapy. *J Neurosurg* 86 (6):943-9. doi:10.3171/jns. 1997.86.6.0943.

Merchant, T. E., Jenkins J. J., Burger P. C., Sanford R. A., Sherwood S. H., Jones-Wallace D., Heideman R. L., Thompson S. J., Helton K. J., and Kun L. E., 2002. Influence of tumor grade on time to progression after irradiation for localized ependymoma in children. *Int J Radiat Oncol Biol Phys* 53 (1):52-7.

Merchant, T. E., Li C., Xiong X., Kun L. E., Boop F. A., and Sanford R. A., 2009. Conformal radiotherapy after surgery for paediatric ependymoma: a prospective study. *Lancet Oncol* 10 (3):258-66.

Nakamura, M., Ishii K., Watanabe K., Tsuji T., Matsumoto M., Toyama Y., and Chiba K., 2009. Long-term surgical outcomes for myxopapillary ependymomas of the cauda equina. *Spine* (Phila Pa 1976) 34 (21):E756-60. doi: 10.1097/BRS.0b013e3181b34d16.

Oya, N., Shibamoto Y., Nagata Y., Negoro Y., and Hiraoka M., 2002. Postoperative radiotherapy for intracranial ependymoma: analysis of prognostic factors and patterns of failure. *J Neurooncol* 56 (1):87-94.

Perilongo, G., Massimino M., Sotti G., Belfontali T., Masiero L., Rigobello L., Garre L., Carli M., Lombardi F., Solero C., Sainati L., Canale V., del Prever A. B., Giangaspero F., Andreussi L., Mazza C., and Madon E., 1997. Analyses of prognostic factors in a retrospective review of 92 children with ependymoma: Italian Pediatric Neuro-Oncology Group. *Med Pediatr Oncol* 29 (2):79-85.

Phi, J. H., Wang K. C., Park S. H., Kim I. H., Kim I. O., Park K. D., Ahn H. S., Lee J. Y., Son Y. J., and Kim S. K., 2012. Pediatric infratentorial ependymoma: prognostic significance of anaplastic histology. *J Neurooncol* 106 (3):619-26. doi: 10.1007/s11060-011-0699-x.

Pollack, I. F., Gerszten P. C., Martinez A. J., Lo K. H., Shultz B., Albright A. L., Janosky J., and Deutsch M., 1995. Intracranial ependymomas of childhood: long-term outcome and prognostic factors. *Neurosurgery* 37 (4):655-66; discussion 666-7.

Preston-Martin, S. 1996, Epidemiology of primary CNS neoplasms. *Neurol Clin* 14 (2):273-90.

Purdy, E., Johnston D. L., Bartels U., Fryer C., Carret A. S., Crooks B., Eisenstat D. D., Lafay-Cousin L., Larouche V., Wilson B., Zelcer S., Silva M., Bouffet E., Keene D., and Strother D. R., 2014. Ependymoma in children under the age of 3 years: a report from the Canadian Pediatric Brain Tumour Consortium. *J Neurooncol* 117 (2):359-64. doi:10.1007/s1 1060-014-1396-3.

Ragel, B. T., Osborn A. G., Whang K., Townsend J. J., Jensen R. L., and Couldwell W. T., 2006. Subependymomas: an analysis of clinical and imaging features. *Neurosurgery* 58 (5):881-90; discussion 881-90. doi:10. 1227/01.NEU.0000209928.04532.09.

Rickert, C. H., and Paulus W. 2001, Epidemiology of central nervous system tumors in childhood and adolescence based on the new WHO classification. *Childs Nerv Syst* 17 (9):503-11. doi:10.1007/s0038101004 96.

Robertson, P. L., Zeltzer P. M., Boyett J. M., Rorke L. B., Allen J. C., Geyer J. R., Stanley P., Li H., Albright A. L., McGuire-Cullen P., Finlay J. L., Stevens K. R., Jr., Milstein J. M., Packer R. J., and Wisoff J., 1998. Survival and prognostic factors following radiation therapy and chemotherapy for ependymomas in children: a report of the Children's Cancer Group. *J Neurosurg* 88 (4):695-703. doi:10.3171/jns.1998.88.4. 0695.

Rodriguez, D., Cheung M. C., Housri N., Quinones-Hinojosa A., Camphausen K., and Koniaris L. G., 2009. Outcomes of malignant CNS ependymomas: an examination of 2408 cases through the Surveillance, Epidemiology, and End Results (SEER) database (1973-2005). *J Surg Res* 156 (2):340-51. doi:10.1016/j.jss.2009.04.024.

Rogers, L., Pueschel J., Spetzler R., Shapiro W., Coons S., Thomas T., and Speiser B., 2005. Is gross-total resection sufficient treatment for posterior fossa ependymomas? *J Neurosurg* 102 (4):629-36. doi:10.3171/jns.2005. 102.4.0629.

Roldan Urgoiti, G. B., Singh A. D., Tsang R. Y., Nordal R. A., Lim G., Chan J. A., Starreveld Y. P., de Robles P. A., Biagioni B. J., Hamilton M. G., and Easaw J. C., 2014. Population based analysis ependymoma patients in alberta from 1975 to 2007. *Can J Neurol Sci* 41 (6):742-7. doi:10.1017/cjn.2014.107.

Rushing, E. J., Cooper P. B., Quezado M., Begnami M., Crespo A., Smirniotopoulos J. G., Ecklund J., Olsen C., and Santi M., 2007. Subependymoma revisited: clinicopathological evaluation of 83 cases. *J Neurooncol* 85 (3):297-305. doi:10.1007/s11060-007-9411-6.

Safaee, M., Oh M. C., Mummaneni P. V., Weinstein P. R., Ames C. P., Chou D., Berger M. S., Parsa A. T., and Gupta N., 2014. Surgical outcomes in spinal cord ependymomas and the importance of extent of resection in children and young adults. *J Neurosurg Pediatr* 13 (4):393-9. doi:10. 3171/2013.12.PEDS13383.

Scheithauer, B. W. 1978. Symptomatic subependymoma. Report of 21 cases with review of the literature. *J Neurosurg* 49 (5):689-96. doi:10.3171/jns. 1978.49.5.0689.

Shirasawa, H., Ishii K., Iwanami A., Mikami S., Toyama Y., Matsumoto M., and Nakamura M., 2014. Pediatric myxopapillary ependymoma treated with subtotal resection and radiation therapy: a case report and review of the literature. *Spinal Cord* 52 Suppl 2:S18-20. doi:10.1038/sc.2014.95.

Timmermann, B., Kortmann R. D., Kuhl J., Meisner C., Slavc I., Pietsch T., and Bamberg M., 2000. Combined postoperative irradiation and chemotherapy for anaplastic ependymomas in childhood: results of the German prospective trials HIT 88/89 and HIT 91. *Int J Radiat Oncol Biol Phys* 46 (2):287-95.

Vaidya, K., Smee R., and Williams J. R., 2012. Prognostic factors and treatment options for paediatric ependymomas. *J Clin Neurosci* 19 (9): 1228-35. doi:10.1016/ j.jocn.2012.02.006.

Villano, J. L., Parker C. K., and Dolecek T. A., 2013. Descriptive epidemiology of ependymal tumours in the United States. *Br J Cancer* 108 (11):2367-71. doi:10.1038/bjc.2013.221.

Zacharoulis, S., and Moreno L., 2009. Ependymoma: an update. *J Child Neurol* 24 (11):1431-8. doi: 10.1177/0883073809339212.

In: Ependymomas
Editor: Raquel Fowler

ISBN: 978-1-63484-405-5

Chapter 3

On the Anaplastic Variant of Ependymoma

Davide Schiffer**, *Laura Annovazzi and Marta Mellai
Research Center/Policlinico di Monza Foundation, Vercelli, Italy

1. Abstract

Anaplastic ependymoma represents a nosographic and epidemiological problem as it has been, and still it is, difficult to distinguish from grade II tumors, and thus its incidence cannot be exactly calculated. The main features required for the tumor recognition are high cell density, high number of mitoses or high Ki-67/MIB-1 labeling index. However, the crucial point is represented by the threshold of the number of mitoses, which in the authors' experience, must exceed 20%.

A true genetic marker for the anaplastic variant is still lacking; however, a small spectrum of genetic aberrations is usually found.

The differential diagnosis of the anaplastic variant *versus* neuroepithelial tumors is not problematic. The only diagnostic critical point is represented by the appearance of anaplasia in *foci* that can escape detection or of an advanced status of anaplasia that hampers the recognition of the tumor as ependymomatous.

In this chapter, prognosis, prognostic factors and survival will be discussed, taking into account that the tumor may have four different locations and may need different surgical treatments. The standard strategy relies on radiation therapy while chemotherapy plays a secondary role. Temozolomide and other drugs are currently employed in clinical trials.

2. Introduction

In the book of the World Health Organization (WHO) classification of tumors of the central nervous system (CNS) [1], as a compendium of literature review and qualified personal experiences, the existence of a malignant ependymoma with an unfavorable course

* Corresponding Author: davide.schiffer@unito.it.

and an adequate histology has been described [2]. Adequate histology corresponds to what happens in gliomas during malignization, i.e., increased cellularity, brisk mitotic activity, microvascular proliferations (MVPs), necroses, etc. However, a strict relationship between histology and outcome is not always found. This is a debated problem among pathologists from the application of a three grade [3–5] or four grade [6, 7] classification system. Currently, the three grade system is widely accepted in the histologic diagnosis of ependymomas, even though the criteria used remains controversial, especially in pediatric tumors [8–14].

In the attempt to identify the anaplastic variant using the same criteria as for gliomas, the frequency of the anaplastic variant in the different series varied from 40 to 94% [15].

As for survival, it has been observed that the anaplastic variant might not show a worse outcome in comparison with other variants [16]. It was already known that the classic subdivision into cellular, epithelial and papillary variants [17] was devoid of any prognostic significance [18, 19], unlike structures as pseudorosettes, canals, rosettes. In a collection of 298 supratentorial cases, no correlation emerged between the diagnosis of the anaplastic variant according to common criteria and survival [20]. Finally, in a subgroup of 173 cases from the same series, the only histopathologic variables significantly correlated with prognosis, among necroses, endothelial proliferation, formation of *glomeruli*, calcifications, microcysts, *pseudopapillae*, lymphocytic infiltration, clear and giant cells, etc., were the high cell density and the number of mitoses >20 × 10 high-power field (HPF). An additional histologic feature constantly encountered in these cases was represented by poorly or incompletely developed pseudorosettes [20].

The above quoted remarks apply to malignant supratentorial tumors in adults. In children, malignant cases prevail among infratentorial tumors [21] where anaplasia most frequently occurs (American Brain Tumor Association, 2015).

2.1. Epidemiology

The incidence of the anaplastic variant is not easy to calculate due to its uncertain definition. Since anaplasia is defined as the reversion of differentiation, cell proliferation becomes its emblem. In ependymoma, the labeling index (LI) of the proliferation marker Ki-67/MIB-1 is highly variable and, until it does not exceed 10-20%, it does not correlate with overall survival (OS), i.e., it does not indicate anaplasia. In the different tumor series, thus, the incidence of the anaplastic variant is variable and it may or may not correlate with OS.

Supratentorial malignant tumors grow near the ventricles or deeply in the white matter, they may involve the *foramen* of Monroe causing *hydrocephalus*, reaching the subarachnoid space and disseminating. Ectopic cortical anaplastic ependymomas are rare [22].

The prevalence of the anaplastic ependymoma in supratentorial location in adults and in *posterior fossa* in children must be taken into account, with the higher frequency of ependymomas in the latter than in the former.

The anaplastic variant may develop as a *de novo* tumor entity or can arise from progression of a lower grade ependymoma.

2.2. Clinical Features

Compared to low-grade ependymomas, the anaplastic variant exhibits a more rapid growth and a more aggressive behavior. It often requires additional treatment after surgery and is associated with an increased risk of recurrence. Grade III ependymoma has an unfavorable outcome [2].

2.3. Neuroradiological Features

At magnetic resonance imaging (MRI), ependymomas generally are T1 hypointense, T2 hyperintense and heterogeneous. Cysts and calcifications may be present. The anaplastic variant typically shows Gadolinium contrast enhancement (Figure 1).

Perfusion MRI generally demonstrates markedly elevated relative cerebral blood volume (rCBV) values and, unlike many other glial neoplasms, poor return to baseline that may be related to fenestrated blood vessels and to an incomplete blood-brain barrier (BBB) [23].

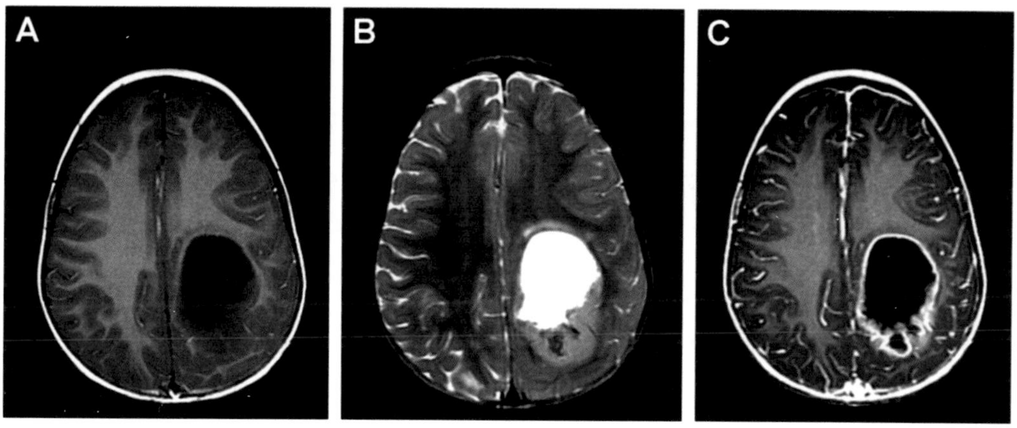

Figure 1. Magnetic resonance imaging (MRI). Anaplastic ependymoma of the right hemisphere in a 23-month-old boy. A – Cystic tumor with a hyperintense border, T1-weighted sequence; B – Diffuse hyperintensity, T2-weighted sequence. C – Contrast enhancement of the borders, T1-weighted sequence after Gadolinium contrast enhancement.

3. Histopathology

At the microscope observation, the anaplastic variant is characterized by highly cellular and poorly differentiated areas with brisk mitotic activity, frequent MVPs and necroses without palisadings. Pseudorosettes are rare and true ependymal rosettes are commonly missing (Figure 2A, B).

The high cell density and high mitotic activity remain the most important diagnostic criteria for anaplasia. Perivascular pseudorosettes may be recognized beside incomplete and poorly developed ones (Figure 2B). Ki-67/MIB-1 LI can be very high, up to or >20% (Figure 2C). Endothelial hyperplasia, MVPs and necroses occur (Figure 2B, D, E) [19, 20].

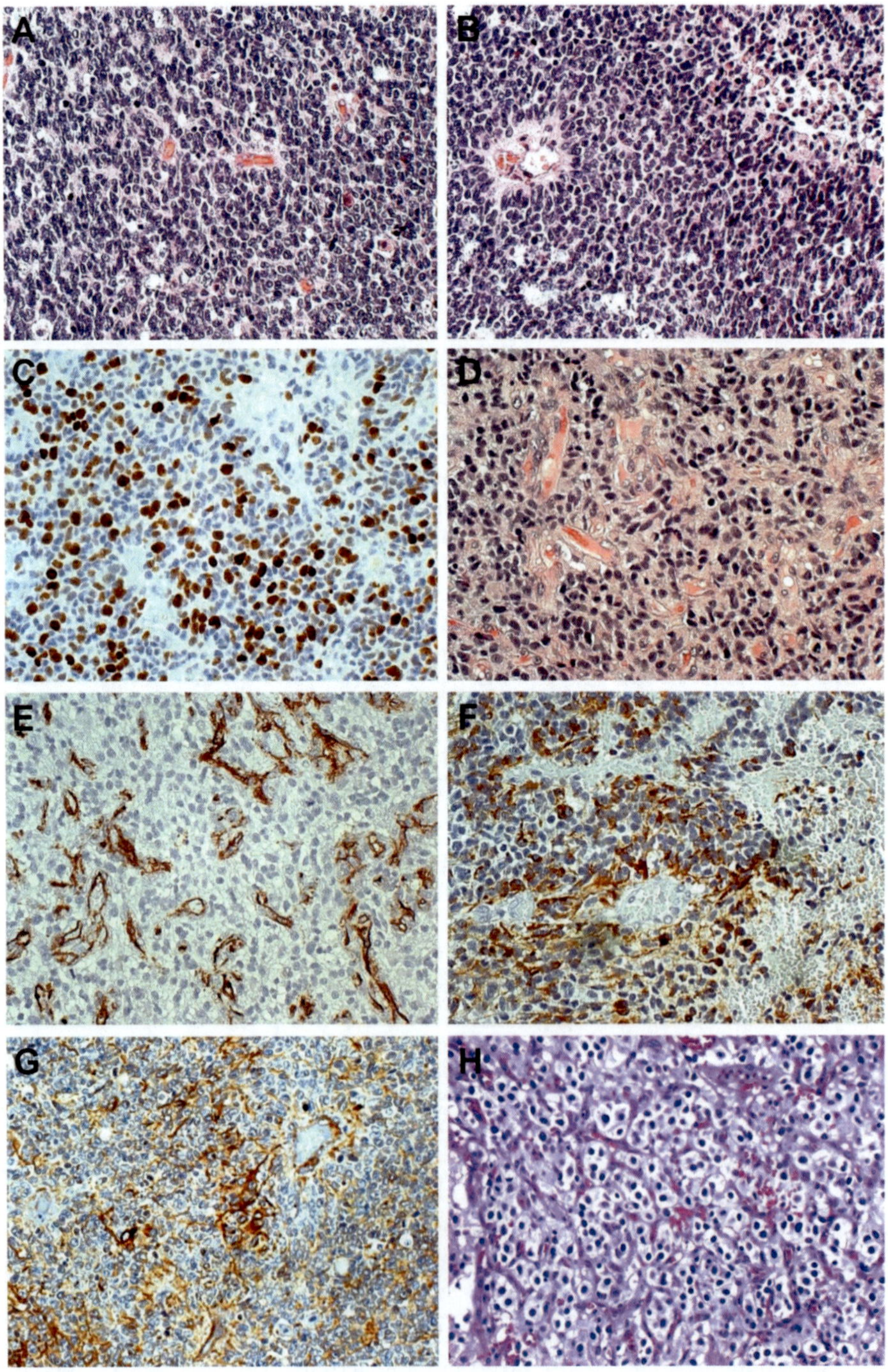

Figure 2. Histopathologic features of anaplastic ependymoma. A – High cell density, several mitoses, nuclear atypias, rosettes and pseudorosettes, H&E,×200; B – Just sketched pseudoresettes and a necrosis in a high proliferative area, H&E, ×200; C – Very high Ki-67/MIB- labeling index, DAB, ×200; D – Endothelial hyperplasia, H&E, ×200; E – Increased density of proliferative vessels, CD34, DAB ×200; F – Rare GFAP-positive cells, especially in pseudorosettes, DAB, ×200; G – Cell clusters positive for Nestin, DAB, ×200; H – Cytoplasmic halo in a clear cell ependymoma, H&E, ×200.

3.1. Immunohistochemistry

Immunohistochemically, the anaplastic variant cannot be distinguished from a grade I or II ependymoma. The expression pattern of glial fibrillary acidic protein (GFAP) and epithelial membrane antigen (EMA) corresponds to that observed in lowgrade tumors, although it is often less pronounced (Figure 2F). In contrast, the LI of the proliferation marker Ki-67/MIB-1 increases up to or >20%. Nestin may be expressed in scattered cells or in small cell clusters (Figure 2G).

The apoptotic index (AI) increases, since it follows the mitotic index (MI) [24]. Increased expression of Tenascin C (TNC), vascular endothelial growth factor (VEGF), epidermal growth factor receptor (EGFR) and p53 has been found, in contrast to a lower expression of cyclin-dependent kinase inhibitor p27/Kip1 and p14^{ARF} [25, 26].

Expression of telomerase reverse transcriptase (TERT) has been found to be increased, as well as its nuclear chaperone Nucleolin [27], and has also been found to be a prognostic factor by multivariate analysis [27, 28]. Members of the receptor tyrosine kinase 1 (RTK1) family have been found to be intensely expressed in highly proliferative adult ependymomas [29] but not in pediatric tumors [26]. Possibly, RTK1 family members behave differently in pediatric and adult tumors.

The threshold of the Ki-67/MIB-1 LI is a very important item. As previously said, it indicates the anaplastic variant when >20% [20]; it has also been found to exceed 25%, also in tumors from the *posterior fossa* [29, 30]. Using lower thresholds, a correlation with survival could not be found [31, 32]. Thus, only a high Ki-67/MIB-1 LI can be considered as a typical feature of anaplasia [27, 33–35].

3.2. Electron Microscopy

Morphological studies by electron microscopy have been applied to the identification of ependymoma variants [36–40].

Some studies focused on the analysis of ciliary structures. In a recent one, it was shown that differentiated ependymomas contain large basal bodies and up to three cilia lacking centrioles. In contrast, the more aggressive anaplastic variant contains neither ependymal nor primary cilia, lacks basal bodies but shows a centrosome formed by two perpendicularly oriented centrioles [41]. Notably, primary cilia have a critical role in neurogenesis since they condition the development of adult neural stem cells [42]. As a matter of fact, cilia and centrosome defects have been associated with a variety of human diseases and neoplasms, including malignant brain tumors [43, 44].

The presence of centrioles in the anaplastic ependymoma represents a peculiar ultrastructure feature useful in the diagnostic practice.

4. Differential Diagnosis

When the typical tumor phenotype is present, the differential diagnosis is not problematic. Mistakes only occur when anaplasia is distributed in small *foci* thus becoming scarcely recognizable. Alternately, anaplasia can be so widespread and advanced that the ependymomatous nature is not more recognizable. In these cases, it could be useful to pay attention to the presence of incomplete and barely detectable perivascular pseudorosettes [20]. This is one of the reasons why, according to some authors, the histologic grading is a subjective factor in patient stratification [45, 46]. Nevertheless, the failure in the diagnosis of the ependymomatous type does not necessarily mean to fail the identification of the histologic grade. The presence of a high cell density and a high MI grants the grade III.

5. Clear Cell Ependymoma

This is a rare variety of ependymoma characterized by sheets of uniform cells with rounded nuclei and encircling perinuclear, clear halos [47, 48] (Figure 2H). It must be distinguished from oligodendrogliomas, central neurocytomas, hemangioblastomas and metastatic renal cell carcinomas and it is characterized by a tendency to recur despite therapy. In a series of 166 ependymomas, ten cases showed features of clear cell ependymoma, corresponding to an incidence of 6%. In seven out of ten tumors, increased cellularity, several mitoses, microvascular hyperplasia and necrosis without pseudopalisading were the histologic signs of malignancy. Immunohisto-chemically, GFAP, EMA and S100 were typically expressed, and in five cases, deletion of DAL-1 and CEP18 were detected by fluorescent *in situ* hybridization (FISH). Median 5-year survival rates for progression-free survival (PFS) and OS were 34% ± 20% and 75% ± 19%, respectively, with a median follow-up of 37 months [49]. This finding means that this tumor variant has a more aggressive behavior compared with other histologic types. However, the most aggressive character of the tumor is probably linked to the occurrence of anaplastic *foci* with a high Ki-67/MIB-1 LI, regardless of the clear cell aspect by itself. As in general in ependymoma, they can become undetectable.

6. Etiology

No clear etiology has been associated with ependymoma to date. An increased incidence of spinal ependymomas has been reported in patients with neurofibromatosis type 2 (NF2) [50]. The NF2 gene is located on chromosome 22q12, which is frequently lost in patients with adult spinal ependymoma [50–53]. However, most of these tumors, in particular those that develop intracranially, do not harbor NF2 mutations. Although the NF2 gene may be involved in the origin of a subgroup of spinal ependymomas, it is probably not the crucial tumor suppressor gene (TSG) on chromosome 22 involved in the tumorigenesis of sporadic intracranial tumors.

Malignant pediatric ependymomas in other types of familial tumor syndromes of the nervous system (i.e., Turcot's syndrome [54] and Li-Fraumeni syndrome [55]) are reported in literature.

Notably, clustering of pediatric and adult ependymomas, including the anaplastic variant, in non NF2-families suggests inheritance of a genetic susceptibility to this tumor type [56–59].

6.1. Molecular Genetics

Cytogenetic studies by karyotyping and comparative genomic hybridization (CGH) techniques described several chromosomal abnormalities in ependymoma. A meta-analysis of all CGH studies on more than 300 primary ependymomas revealed that pediatric and adult tumors are biologically different entities [26, 60]. This finding suggests that ependymomas are heterogeneous and can be classified as distinct tumor subtypes based on patient age, tumor location, and genetic profiles [61–63].

Interestingly, 50% of tumors are characterized by a balanced genomic profile. A balanced profile with, at least, focal partial chromosomal imbalances (median 3.8 *per* tumor) prevails in pediatric tumors, while adult tumors typically show several broad chromosomal imbalances (median 7.5 *per* tumor). With regard to the anaplastic variant, a recent study revealed a low frequency of chromosomal imbalances (median 2 *per* tumor) [64]. Remarkably, the rate of cytogenetic imbalances in ependymoma is inversely correlated with the histologic malignancy grade [64, 65].

6.2. Cytogenetic Aberrations

The most commonly identified chromosomal aberrations in ependymoma include copy number gain on 1q21-32, loss of chromosomes 22q, 6q and 9p; gain on chromosome 7q is exclusively associated with spinal tumors [66–69]. Location-specific cytogenetic aberrations in intracranial *versus* spinal tumors may refer to the different tumor locations observed in children and adults.

Cytogenetic data on the anaplastic variant are scarce and no exclusive genetic aberrations have been reported. However, gain on chromosome 1q21-32 and loss of chromosomes 1p, 6q, 9p and 14q are preferentially associated with this histologic variant [66, 69–71].

Based on the CGH meta-analysis, the most common genomic aberration in both primary and recurrent pediatric intracranial tumors is a copy number gain of chromosome 1q21-32 with an incidence of approximately 25% [26, 70, 71]. Gain on 1q is detected in grade II and III tumors, preferentially in infratentorial/*posterior fossa* tumors in children [64] and is strongly associated with anaplastic histologic features, tumor aggressiveness, and poor outcome [26, 65, 66, 68, 70–75].

Then, based on these findings, the chromosome 1 should contain candidate genes involved in ependymoma tumorigenesis and progression, as well as in resistance to therapeutic treatment. Efforts have been made to identify the critical region and the crucial genes. Two minimal gained regions have been identified at the chromosomal *loci* 1q21.3-23.1 and 1q21.1-32.1, the latter significantly correlated with tumor recurrence [26, 68, 69, 72, 76]. Notably, gain on 1q25 has been identified as independent prognostic marker for significantly lower PFS and OS [68].

The dual-specificities phosphatase 12 (DUSP12) gene at 1q23.3 has been proposed as a driver oncogene for the anaplastic ependymoma since its over-expression has been associated with more aggressive tumors [68]. DUSP12 is involved in the cell cycle control and potentially in the malignant transformation [68, 77]. It also plays a role for the cell survival in response to heat shock-induced cell death [78]. Potential driver oncogenes located within the hot spot region 1q21-32 include laminin, PRELP, HSPA6 (1q32), GAC1, CHI3L1 (1q32.1), TPR, JTB, SHC1, S100A10 (1q21) and other S100 family members [26, 79–82].

Importantly, the gain on 1q is typically associated with an unfavorable outcome in neuroblastoma, Wilms' tumor, and Ewing's sarcoma, suggesting a common role in pediatric tumor initiation, progression, and recurrence [83–85].

Loss of chromosome 6q is commonly detected in infratentorial tumors, including recurrences, whereas deletions on chromosome 9 occur more frequently in supratentorial tumors [65, 66, 73, 76, 86]. Hot spots of deletion have been identified by loss of heterozygosity (LOH) analysis at 6q15-16, 6q21-22.1 and 6q24.3-25.3, subsequently limited to 6q24.3 and 6q25.2-25.3 [67, 87]. Remarkably, loss of 6q25.3 is a favorable prognostic marker for OS in patients with intracranial anaplastic ependymomas. Inactivation of sortin nexin 9 (SNX9) and synaptojanin 2 (SYNJ2) genes, both located at 6q25.3 and involved in the regulation of cell migration and invasion, may inhibit tumor progression [87]. Additional putative TSGs in these regions, such as the polyamine biosynthesis gene (AMD1) and the cyclin-dependent kinase (CDK11) both at 6q21, and SASH1 at 6q24.3 have been reported to be down-regulated [80].

With regard to the chromosome 9, which is frequently deleted in ependymoma, a homozygous deletion of the CDKN2A*locus* at 9p21.3 has been reported and typically associated with anaplastic tumors [61, 68, 75, 88]. Consistent with this finding, a decreased expression of the $p14^{ARF}$ protein was significantly associated with tumor aggressiveness [25]. Two regions at 9p21.2-22.3 and at 9q31.3-33.2 resulted as the most commonly deleted regions in both adult and pediatric ependymomas. Candidate TSGs located within 9q31.3-33.2 include DBC1, markedly down-regulated in bladder cancer and gliomas [89, 90]. Loss of chromosome 9 has also been implicated in the development of clear cell ependymomas [91].

In contrast, gains on 9q33-34, covering NOTCH1 and TNC, are common in recurrent tumors, suggesting the involvement of both oncogenes in the progression of pediatric ependymomas with *posterior fossa* location [76]. In this regard, inhibition of NOTCH pathway by a γ-secretase inhibitor may hamper the growth of ependymoma stem cell cultures [76]. Moreover, gene amplification on 9qter increases after subsequent recurrences, more frequently in older children [76].

Loss of chromosomes 1p and 14q prevails in recurrences and tumor metastasis with a significantly increasing extent in relation to the distance from the site of local recurrence to metastasis [91].

Monosomy of the chromosome 10 was reported in few cases (4/17, 23.6%) of infratentorial anaplastic ependymomas [52, 65] in association with LOH of 17p13 [65]. Mutations of the TP53 were only occasionally detected [51].

6.3. Timing

The stepwise accumulation of the distinct molecular events during the progression from a low-grade tumor has been clarified in a patient, 18-years of age, affected by supratentorial anaplastic and progressively metastasizing ependymoma [91]. Genome-wide copy number analysis on the primary tumor, first and second local recurrence and subcutaneous metastasis, revealed monosomy of chromosome 9 and homozygous deletion of the CDKN2A *locus* in the primary tumor and sequential deletions on chromosomes 1 (1p36.32-1p36.22) and 14

(14q32.32-14q12) in both recurrences and metastasis. Gradual loss at 1p36 was associated with loss of protein expression of the putative TSG AJAP1/SHREW1 on 1p36.32 [91]. This gene is located within the chromosomal region (1p36.32-1p36.22) lost in the transition from localized to metastatic disease and is involved in cell adhesion, cell motility and tumor invasion in oligodendroglioma [91–95]. The absence of gain on 1q is in line with the finding that it is less common in intracranial compared to spinal ependymomas [64, 66].

The finding of a homozygous deletion of the CDKN2A *locus* ($p16^{INK4A}$) emphasizes its role in the ependymoma tumorigenesis and further supports CDKN2A as a key player in tumor initiation [68]. The sequential deletions on chromosomes 1p and 14q detected in local recurrences and metastasis additionally indicate candidate genes involved in tumor progression and/or metastasis.

6.4. Epigenetics

Aberrant promoter hypermethylation of CpG islands is a peculiar feature of several cancers. A genome-wide epigenomic profiling in ependymomas [96] identified a hypermethylator phenotype similar to the "CpG island hypermethylator phenotype" (CIMP) that was previously identified in gliomas, acute myeloid leukemia (AML) and colon cancers [97–100]. The CIMP prevails in supratentorial and spinal pediatric ependymomas if compared with *posterior fossa* tumors and is characterized by aberrant methylation of candidate TSGs involved in the control of cell growth and apoptosis, as well as in the immune system (including members of the JNK pathway, PPARG and RASSF1A) [96]. RASSF1A, an effector of Ras, has been found to be the most frequently hypermethylated TSG, described in up to 86% of ependymomas of all histologic subtypes [96, 101]. Down-regulation of RASSF1A results in loss of cell cycle control, enhanced genetic instability and resistance to k-Ras and tumor necrosis α (TNF α)-induced apoptosis [102]. Other commonly hypermethylated genes in ependymoma include HIC1 in 83% of intracranial tumors [103], CDKN2A ($p16^{INK4A}$) in 21% of supratentorial tumors [63, 75], CDKN2B ($p15^{INK4B}$) and CDKN2A ($p14^{ARF}$) in 32 and 33% of tumors, respectively [104]. Aberrant methylation of the O^6-methylguanine-DNA methyltransferase (MGMT) gene was generally found at a lower rate and not in recurrent anaplastic tumors [105].

The difference in the global level of methylation varies according to the tumor location in the CNS and supports epigenetic silencing of TSGs as an important mechanism in the pathogenesis of supratentorial and spinal, but not *posterior fossa,* ependymomas [96].

Unlike gliomas, the CIMP was not associated with survival in ependymoma or in pediatric *posterior fossa* tumors [93, 96]. However, CIMP-positive *posterior fossa* tumors of childhood are responsive to clinical drugs targeting DNA or H3K27 methylation both *in vitro* and *in vivo* [93].

A diagnostic classifier tool based on DNA methylation profiles, named MethPed, was recently developed to identify pediatric brain tumor subtypes, including ependymoma [106].

6.5. Gene Expression Profiling

The comparison of gene expression profiling data between low *versus* high grade tumors and between primary *versus* recurrent tumors revealed heterogeneous results that are very scarce for the anaplastic variant [62, 107, 108].

Compared to low-grade tumors, grade III ependymomas show up-regulation of genes involved in the Wnt/β-catenin signaling activation, cell cycle/proliferation regulation (Cyclin B2/D1/G2, cyclin-dependent kinases CDK2/4/5, cell division cycle proteinsCDC25A/ 25B,25C/2, and minimal chromosome maintenance proteins MCM2/3/4/5/6/7), apoptosis (tumor necrosis factor super family members TNFRSF11A/21 and caspases CASP1/4), angiogenesis (VEGF, VEGFR2, VEGFB, TNIP2 and DOC2), and remodeling of adherent junctions through E-cadherin destruction (MET, MN23H1, caveolin, RAB5/7 GTPases). The Wnt signaling activation in grade III ependymomas has been proved by the up-regulation of Wnt ligand (Wnt11), frizzled receptors (FZD2/5/8), disheveled (DVL2/3) and β-catenin encoding (CTNNB1) genes [62, 107, 108].

According to distinct gene expression profiling, three independent studies proved the existence of at least two genetically and biologically distinct variants of infratentorial/ *posterior fossa* ependymomas [63, 109, 110]. They were defined as Group A (Group 1 according to Wani et al. [110]) and Group B (Group 2according to Wani et al. [110]) [109]. Tumors belonging to Group A are associated with a poor outcome, and recur at a significantly higher rate and develop metastasis in >80% of the cases. They do not display large cytogenetic aberrations and are characterized by a classic cancer-related signature (EGFR, platelet-derived growth factor [PDGF], VEGF and mitogen-activated protein kinase [MAPK]). In contrast, tumors belonging to Group B show large chromosomal aberrations, affecting total deletion of either the p- or q- chromosomal arm or the entire chromosome. They display a specific over-expression of genes implicated in ciliogenesis, microtubule assembly and mitochondrial metabolism [109]. A 10-gene signature has also been validated by Wani and co-authors to reliably classify *posterior fossa* tumors in the two mentioned groups in the clinical practice and to stratify patients for therapeutic purposes [110].

A third study by Johnson and colleagues on 83 ependymomas with supra- and infratentorial locations identified nine molecular subgroups mainly based on tumor location. They include four supratentorial subgroups (A-D), two subgroups of *posterior fossa* tumors, including spinal ependymomas (E, F), and three subgroups of exclusively *posterior fossa* tumors [63].

7. Survival and Prognosis

More than half of ependymomas occur in children; ninety percent are intracranial and two thirds of these are located in the *posterior fossa*. They may share characteristics with germ cell tumors and can occur in the sacrococcygeal region, mediastinum and ovary (see ependymomas in familial syndromes) [111–113]. For different locations and patient age, pediatric tumors must be considered separately from the adult ones.

Pediatric tumors show a median 5-year survival rate from 39% to 64% with a median 5-year PFS rate from 23% to 45% [114]. Late recurrences up to 15 years may occur [115]. The worst prognosis is observed in children <3 years of age and with *posterior fossa* tumors [116], but it is unclear whether this is due to their malignancy or to their location and age.

Ependymomas in adults are rather rare, accounting for only 3% of all primary CNS tumors. Spinal ependymomas prevail in adults and *posterior fossa* tumors in children, whereas supratentorial ependymomas are more evenly distributed between adults and children.

The identification of prognostic markers and the relationship between patient outcome and tumor grade are controversial [45, 115–118]. Generally, pediatric ependymomas have a worse prognosis compared to adults [2].

As said before, several studies described an association between anaplasia and poor outcome or between the former and outcome after radiotherapy [116, 118], whereas others did not accept such association.

Two independent studies, including a meta-analysis on 2,408 ependymomas, demonstrated that the tumor grade is an independent prognostic marker for PFS [119, 120], but not for OS in *posterior fossa* tumors [45]. A novel histopathologic grading scheme was elaborated after the evaluation of 229 intracranial tumors by five neuropathologists from European clinical trials of infants (SFOP/CNS9204) and older children (AEIOP/CNS9904). Cell density, mitotic activity, and angiogenesis indicated important features for classification of grade II and III tumors. However, a significant association between the tumor grade and PFS was only found in one trial (AEIOP) related to older children [121]. This is in agreement with the evidence that only high values of cell density and mitotic activity can indicate the anaplastic variant [20, 29, 30].

In our experience, a number of mitoses >20 × 10 HPF (Figure 3A) and the presence of necroses (Figure 3B) are significant prognostic factors ($p < 0.05$ for both) in supratentorial ependymomas by univariate survival analysis [19]. Mitoses ($p < 0.0005$), cell density ($p < 0.005$) and age at diagnosis >16 ($p < 0.05$) remain significant prognostic factors in supratentorial ependymomas after multivariate survival analysis [19]. Moreover, the anaplastic histology correlates with OS not when diagnosed with common criteria (Figure 3C) but only according to the number of mitoses (Figure 3D) [19, 20].

Recently, tumor grade and brain location have been associated to worse PFS and OS by univariate analysis [122]. The Ki-67/MIB-1 LI was dichotomized and patients were subdivided in two groups according to a Ki-67/MIB-1 LI > or ≤ 10%. The risk of death and recurrence were respectively 3.5 and 4.7 times greater in the former than in the latter. In particular, patients with a brain tumor, rather than a spinal lesion, and a high Ki-67/MIB-1 LI have a higher death risk. In conclusion, the Ki-67/MIB-1 LI conditions a shorter PFS for the overall group and even more for the anaplastic variant [122].

Currently, extent of tumor resection, metastatic status, and WHO grading are widely accepted as the main factors for patient stratification [120], although authors have questioned the objectivity of the histologic diagnosis [45, 123]. Prognostic immunohistochemical markers would include TNC [109], Nestin [91], TERT [27, 28], neurofilament light polypeptide 70 (NEFL) [124] LAMA2 and NELL2 [109, 110]. In grade III tumors, immunoreactivity for p53, TNC, VEGF, and EGFR have been associated with decreased PFS [69, 91].

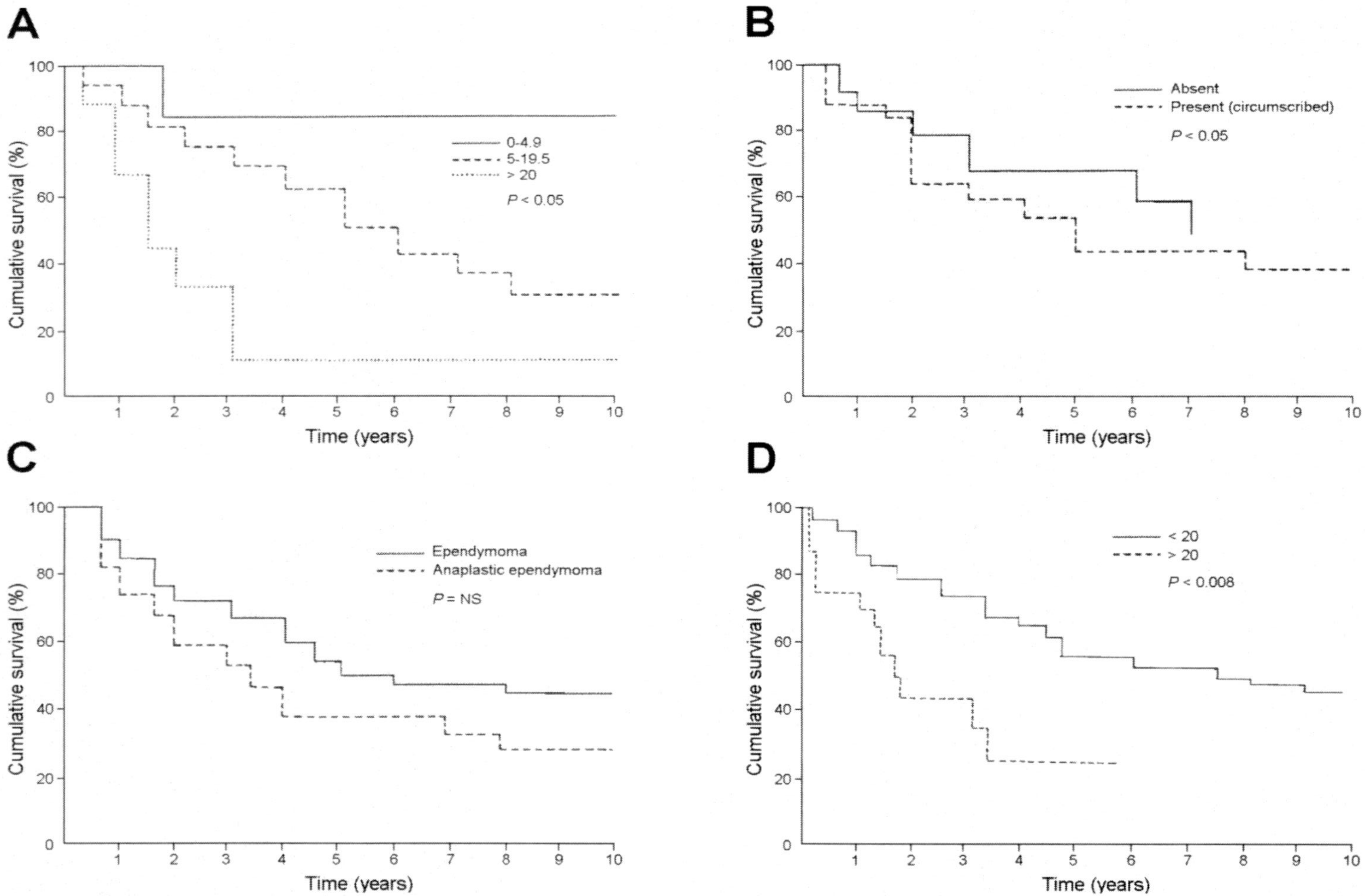

Figure 3. Univariate survival analysis by the Kaplan-Meier method in supratentorial ependymomas. A – Significant correlation between overall survival (OS) and the number of mitoses; B – Significant correlation between OS and the presence of necroses; C – Lack of correlation between OS and the anaplastic histology when diagnosed with common criteria; D – Statistically significant correlation between OS and the anaplastic histology when diagnosed according to a number of mitoses >20 × 10 HPF [19, 20].

According to the molecular asset, a staging system has been proposed by Korshunov and co-authors for standard, intermediate and high genetic risk intracranial ependymomas consisting of three prognostic subgroups. Group 1 (5-year OS of 100%) is characterized by gain on chromosome 9, 15q or 18 and loss of chromosome 6, without gain on 1q or CDKN2A deletion, Group 2 (5-year OS of 78%) by a balanced genomic profile for chromosomes 1q, 6, 9, 15q and 18, without homozygous deletion of CDKN2A, while Group 3 (5-year OS of 32%) is characterized by gain on chromosome 1q or homozygous deletion of the CDKN2A [75], as confirmed later [125, 126]. Cytogenetic aberrations of the Group 3, i.e., gain on 1q25 and homozygous deletion of the CDKN2A *locus*, are associated with the anaplastic variant and are the most powerful independent factors of poor prognosis. In contrast, gains on chromosomes 9q34, 15q22, 18q21 and loss of chromosome 6q23 are associated with a significantly better OS [75]. Loss of 6q25.3 is also prognostic in anaplastic tumors [77].

Gain on 1q25 was recently confirmed as an independent predictor of tumor progression across three independent clinical trials (Children's Cancer Leukemia Group/International Society for Pediatric Oncology [CCLG/SIOP], CNS9204, BBSFOP adjuvant chemotherapy, and primary postoperative radiotherapy [SIOP CNS9904]) [125]. In conclusion, copy number gain on 1q is the most widely reported negative prognostic molecular marker for both supra- and infratentorial tumors.

A cluster of microRNAs (miRNAs) (let-7d, miR-596 and miR-367) on chromosome 1q42 has been significantly associated with OS. Moreover, miR-203 is an independent marker for time to relapse [127].

On the existence of a prognostic gene expression signature in *posterior fossa* ependymomas has been already discussed [109, 110].

8. Treatment

The current management of ependymomas includes surgery or radiosurgery, radiation therapy and adjuvant therapy. According to the National Comprehensive Cancer Network guidelines for adults (NCCN, 2015), after gross-total resection (GTR) of an intracranial grade II tumor, limited field fractionated external beam radiation therapy (LFFEBRT) is considered at variance with the "wait and see" approach. In case of subtotal resection (STR), diagnosis of a grade III tumor or a second relapse, radiation therapy is recommended. For children <3 years, chemotherapy is fostered to avoid adverse neurocognitive effects caused by radiation [128]. In older children and adults, radiotherapy is the standard treatment after resection for most patients with grade II ependymoma.

By retrospective data on 182 intracranial pediatric patients, the best PFS rate and OS result after GTR. Patients with grade II tumors have better OS after GTR+EBRT and better PFS after GTR alone, whereas patients with grade III tumors have a better OS after STR+EBRT. The same effect on PFS is observed in patients affected by infratentorial tumors [129].

For primary spinal anaplastic ependymomas, GTR and adjuvant radiotherapy significantly prolong PFS and OS, but chemotherapy with temozolomide (TMZ), cisplatin and teniposide does not [130]. However, TMZ has been successfully used in the treatment of pediatric refractory anaplastic ependymomas with low MGMT expression [131].

Interestingly, in a case of cerebellar cavernoma treated with stereotactic gamma knife surgery (GKS), an anaplastic ependymoma developed with dissemination into the lateral ventricles [132]. Since the tumor displayed aberrant promoter methylation of the MGMT gene, the patient was adjuvantly treated with TMZ-based chemotherapy according to the EORTC/NCIC-regimen published by Stupp et al. [133]. Sixteen days after the TMZ initiation, no trace of the residual tumor was visible [132].

Postoperative chemotherapy with TMZ has been also used as salvage treatment for recurrent intracranial adult ependymomas with responses from both grade II and III tumors [134].

Methotrexate directly administered into the fourth ventricle in children with malignant ependymoma was employed in a pilot clinical trial [135]. The last therapeutic tool in the treatment of pediatric intracranial ependymomas, including malignant tumors, is proton radiation (PRT) after re-irradiation that has been demonstrated to be efficacious [136]. Imetelstat, a phase 2 telomerase inhibitor, abolishes tumorigenicity of pediatric ependymoma tumor initiating cells (TICs) [137]. Finally, epigenetic modifiers such as inhibitors of DNA methylation (decitabine) and histone deacetylation (vorinostat) may also be considered as a rationale and potential therapeutic tool [138, 139].

The therapy is, however, in continuous refining as new biomarkers or predictive factors are described and as more of them will be discovered, more therapies can become individualized.

Conclusion

The diagnosis of ependymoma is mainly based on histologic and immunohistochemical criteria. In the diagnosis, the crucial point is to separate grade II and III tumors. The high number of mitoses is the most useful criterion, beside the finding of poor and incomplete perivascular pseudorosettes. Electron microscopy may improve routine diagnosis by supporting the identification of critical epithelial features.

Prognosis, prognostic factors, and survival are adequate for a grade III tumor. From the therapeutic point of view, the extent of surgical removal and radiotherapy are the most important factors. Chemotherapy plays a secondary role, although clinical trials with TMZ and other drugs are currently in progress.

Acknowledgment

We thank Dr. Maria Consuelo Valentini (Neuroradiology Department/Città della Salute e della Scienza Hospital, Turin, Italy) for providing the MRI figures.

Disclosure of Potential Conflicts of Interest: Authors declare no potential conflicts of interest.

REFERENCES

[1] Louis, DN; Ohgaki, H; Wiestler, OD; Cavenee, WK. *WHO Classification of Tumours of the Central Nervous System* (4th edition). Lyon, France: International Agency for Research on Cancer (IARC); 2007.

[2] McLendon, RE; Wiestler, OD; Kros, JM; Ng, HK. Anaplastic ependymoma. In: Louis, DN; Ohgaki, H; Wiestler, OD; Cavenee, WK, Eds. *WHO Classification of Tumours of the Central Nervous System* (4th edition). Lyon, France: International Agency for Research on Cancer (IARC); 2007; 79-80.

[3] Ringertz, N; Reymond, A. Ependymomas and choroid plexus papillomas. *Journal of Neuropathology and Experimental Neurology*, 1949 8, 355-380.

[4] Goutelle, A; Fisher G. Les ependymomes intracreniens et intrarachidiens. *Neurochirurgie*, 1977 23, 1-236.

[5] Afra, D; Müller, W; Slowik, F; Wilcke, O; Budka, H; Turoczy, L. Supratentorial lobar ependymomas: reports on the grading and survival periods in 80 cases, including 46 recurrences. *Acta Neurochirurgica*, 1983 69, 243-251.

[6] Kernohan, JW; Mabon, RF; Swien, JH; Adson, AW. A simplified classification of the gliomas. *Proceedings of the staff meetings. Mayo Clinic*, 1949 24, 71-75.

[7] Shaw, EG; Evans, RG; Scheithauer, BW; Ilstrup, DM; Earle, JD. Postoperative radiotherapy of intracranial ependymoma in pediatric and adult patients. *International journal of radiation oncology, biology, physics*, 1987 13, 1457-1462.

[8] Mork, SJ; Loken, AC. Ependymoma: a follow-up study of 101 cases. *Cancer*, 1977 40, 907-915.

[9] Ilgren, EB; Stiller, CA; Hughes, JT; Silberman, D; Steckel, N; Kaye, A. Ependymomas: a clinical and pathologic study. Part II. Survival features. *Clinical Neuropathology*, 1984 3, 122-127.

[10] Rawlings, CE 3rd; Giangaspero, F; Burger, PC; Bullard, DE. Ependymomas: a clinicopathologic study. *Surgical Neurology*, 1988 29, 271-281.

[11] Schiffer, D; Chiò, A; Cravioto, H; Giordana, MT; Palma, L; Soffietti, R; Tribolo, A; Vigliani, MC. Ependymomas of childhood: pathological study of 100 cases for survival analysis (abstract). *Pediatric Neuroscience*, 1989 14, 149.

[12] Reni, M; Gatta, G; Mazza, E; Vecht, C. Ependymoma. *Critical Reviews in Oncology/Hematology*, 2007 63, 81-89.

[13] Armstrong, TS; Vera-Bolanos, E; Bekele, BN; Aldape, K; Gilbert, MR. Adult ependymal tumors: prognosis and the M. D. Anderson Cancer Center experience. *Neuro-Oncology*, 2010 12, 862-870.

[14] Warren, K. Ependymomas. The Childhood Brain Tumor Foundation, National Cancer Institute for Neurologic Disorder and Stroke. Germantown, MD, USA. www.childhoodbraintumor.org.

[15] West, CR; Bruce, DA; Duffner, PK. Ependymomas. Factors in clinical and diagnostic staging. *Cancer*, 1985 56, 1812-1816.

[16] Ross, GW; Rubinstein, LJ. Lack of histopathological correlation of malignant ependymomas with postoperative survival. *Journal of Neurosurgery*, 1989 70, 31-36.

[17] Zülch, KJ. Biologie and Pathologie der Hirngeschwulste. *Handbuch der Neurochirurgie* (vol III). Berlin Göttingen Heidelberg, Germany: Springer; 1956.

[18] Rorke, LB. Relationship of morphology of ependymoma in children to prognosis. *Progress in experimental tumor research*, 1987 30, 170-174.

[19] Schiffer, D; Chiò, A; Giordana, MT; Migheli, A; Palma, L; Pollo, B; Soffietti, R; Tribolo, A. Histologic prognostic factors in ependymoma. *Childs Nervous System*, 1991 7, 177-182.

[20] Schiffer, D; Chiò, A; Cravioto, H; Giordana, MT; Migheli, A; Soffietti, R; Vigliani, MC. Ependymoma: internal correlations among pathological signs: the anaplastic variant. *Neurosurgery*, 1991 29, 206-210.

[21] Nazar, GB; Hoffman, HJ; Becker, LE; Jenkin, D; Humphreys, RP; Hendrick, EB. Infratentorial ependymomas in childhood: prognostic factors and treatment. *Journal of Neurosurgery*, 1990 72, 408-417.

[22] Zhang, J; Sai, K; Wang, J; Chen, YS; Yan, SM; Chen, ZP. Ectopic cortical anaplastic ependymoma: an unusual case report and literature review. *Clinical Neurology and Neurosurgery*, 2014 124, 142-145.

[23] Yuh, EL; Barkovich, AJ; Gupta, N. Imaging of ependymomas: MRI and CT. *Childs Nervous System*, 2009 25, 1203-1213.

[24] Schiffer, D; Cavalla, P; Migheli, A; Chiò, A; Giordana, MT; Marino, S; Attanasio, A. Apoptosis and cell proliferation in human neuroepithelial tumors. *Neuroscience Letters*, 1995 195, 81-84.

[25] Korshunov, A; Golanov, A; Timirgaz, V. p14ARF protein (FL-132) immunoreactivity in intracranial ependymomas and its prognostic significance: an analysis of 103 cases. *Acta Neuropathologica*, 2001 102, 271-277.

[26] Kilday, JP; Rahman, R; Dyer, S; Ridley, L; Lowe, J; Coyle, B; Grundy, R. Pediatric ependymoma: biological perspectives. *Molecular Cancer Research*, 2009 7, 765-786.

[27] Ridley, L; Rahman, R; Brundler, MA; Ellison, D; Lowe, J; Robson, K; Prebble, E; Luckett, I; Gilbertson, RJ; Parkes, S; Rand, V; Coyle, B; Grundy, RG; Children's Cancer and Leukaemia Group Biological Studies Committee. Multifactorial analysis of predictors of outcome in pediatric intracranial ependymoma. *Neuro-Oncology*, 2008 10, 675-689.

[28] Tabori, U; Ma, J; Carter, M; Zielenska, M; Rutka, J; Bouffet, E; Bartels, U; Malkin, D; Hawkins, C. Human telomere reverse transcriptase expression predicts progression and survival in pediatric intracranial ependymoma. *Journal of Clinical Oncology*, 2006 24, 1522-1528.

[29] Gilbertson, RJ; Bentley, L; Hernan, R; Junttila, TT; Frank, AJ; Haapasalo, H; Connelly, M; Wetmore, C; Curran, T; Elenius, K; Ellison, DW. ERBB receptor signaling promotes ependymoma cell proliferation and represents a potential novel therapeutic target for this disease. *Clinical Cancer Research*, 2002 8, 3054-3064.

[30] Bennetto, L; Foreman, N; Harding, B; Hayward, R; Ironside, J; Love, S; Ellison, D. Ki-67 immunolabelling index is a prognostic indicator in childhood posterior fossa ependymomas. *Neuropathology and applied neurobiology*,1998 24, 434-440.

[31] Asai, A; Hoshino, T; Edwards, MS; Davis, RL. Predicting the recurrence of ependymomas from the bromodeoxyuridine labeling index. *Childs Nervous System*,1992 8, 273-278.

[32] Zamecnik, J; Snuderl, M; Eckschlager, T; Chanova, M; Hladikova, M; Tichy, M; Kodet, R. Pediatric intracranial ependymomas: prognostic relevance of histological,

immunohistochemical, and flow cytometric factors. *Modern Pathology*, 2003 16, 980-991.

[33] Rushing, EJ; Brown, DF; Hladik, CL; Risser, RC; Mickey, BE; White, CL 3rd. Correlation of bcl-2, p53, and MIB-1 expression with ependymoma grade and subtype. *Modern Pathology*, 1998 11, 464-470.

[34] Suzuki, S; Oka, H; Kawano, N; Tanaka, S; Utsuki, S; Fujii, K. Prognostic value of Ki-67 (MIB-1) and p53 in ependymomas. *Brain Tumor Pathology*, 2001 18, 151-154.

[35] Suri, VS; Tatke, M; Singh, D; Sharma, A. Histological spectrum of ependymomas and correlation of p53 and Ki-67 expression with ependymoma grade and subtype. *Indian Journal of Cancer*, 2004 41, 66-71.

[36] Cenacchi, G; Giangaspero, F; Cerasoli, S; Manetto, V; Martinelli, GN. Ultrastructural characterization of oligodendroglial-like cells in central nervous system tumors. *Ultrastructural Pathology*, 1996 20, 537-547.

[37] Min, KW; Scheithauer, BW. In Clear cell ependymoma: a mimic of oligodendroglioma: clinicopathologic and ultrastructural considerations. *The American journal of surgical pathology*, 1997 21, 820-826.

[38] Lehman, NL. Patterns of brain infiltration and secondary structure formation in supratentorial ependymal tumors. *Journal of Neuropathology and Experimental Neurology*, 2008 67, 900-910.

[39] Jain, D; Sharma, MC; Arora, R; Sarkar, C; Suri, V. Clear cell ependymoma: a mimicker of oligodendroglioma-report of three cases. *Neuropathology*, 2008 28, 366-371.

[40] Fukudome, N; Ohno, E; Mochizuki, M; Eguchi, H; Kojima, H. Three-dimensional reconstructive analysis of intracytoplasmiclumina found in ependymomas. *Rinsho Byori, The Japanese Journal of Clinical Pathology*, 2009 57, 345-350.

[41] Alfaro-Cervelló, C; Soriano-Navarro, M; Ramírez, M; Bernet, L; Martinez Banaclocha, M; Cano, R; Reyes Santías, RM; Forteza-Vila, J; García-Verdugo, JM. Ultrastructural pathology of anaplastic and grade II ependymomas reveals distinctive ciliary structures-electron microscopy redux. *Ultrastructural Pathology*, 2015 39, 23-29.

[42] Han, YG; Spassky, N; Romaguera-Ros, M; Garcia-Verdugo, JM; Aguilar, A; Schneider-Maunoury, S; Alvarez-Buylla, A. Hedgehog signaling and primary cilia are required for the formation of adult neural stem cells. *Nature Neuroscience*, 2008 11, 277-284.

[43] Nigg, EA; Raff, JW. Centrioles, centrosomes, and cilia in health and disease. *Cell*, 2009 139, 663-678.

[44] Han, YG; Kim, HJ; Dlugosz, AA; Ellison, DW; Gilbertson, RJ; Alvarez-Buylla, A. Dual and opposing roles of primary cilia in medulloblastoma development. *Nature Medicine*, 2009 15, 1062-1065.

[45] Tihan, T; Zhou, T; Holmes, E; Burger, PC; Ozuysal, S; Rushing, EJ. The prognostic value of histological grading of posterior fossa ependymomas in children: a Children's Oncology Group study and a review of prognostic factors. *Modern Pathology*, 2008 21, 165-177.

[46] Messahel, B; Ashley, S; Saran, F; Ellison, D; Ironside, J; Phipps, K; Cox, T; Chong, WK; Robinson, K; Picton, S; Pinkerton, CR; Mallucci, C; Macarthur, D; Jaspan, T; Michalski, A; Grundy, RG; Children's Cancer Leukaemia Group Brain Tumour Committee. Relapsed intracranial ependymoma in children in the UK: patterns of

relapse, survival and therapeutic outcome. *European Journal of Cancer*, 2009 45, 1815-1823.

[47] Kawano, N; Yada, K; Yagishita, S. Clear cell ependymoma. A histological variant with diagnostic implications. *Virchows Archiv. A, Pathological anatomy and histopathology*, 1989 415, 467-472.

[48] Burger, PC; Scheithauer, BW. *Tumors of Nervous System.* Washington (United States of America): Armed Forces Institute of Pathology; 1994.

[49] Fouladi, M; Helton, K; Dalton, J; Gilger, E; Gajjar, A; Merchant, T; Kun, L; Newsham, I; Burger, P; Fuller, C. Clear cell ependymoma: a clinicopathologic and radiographic analysis of 10 patients. *Cancer*, 2003 98, 2232-2244.

[50] Rubio, MP; Correa, KM; Ramesh, V; MacCollin, MM; Jacoby, LB; von Deimling, A; Gusella, JF; Louis, DN. Analysis of the neurofibromatosis 2 gene in human ependymomas and astrocytomas. *Cancer Research*, 1994 54, 45-47.

[51] von Haken, MS; White, EC; Daneshvar-Shyesther, L; Sih, S; Choi, E; Kalra, R; Cogen, PH. Molecular genetic analysis of chromosome arm 17p and chromosome arm 22q DNA sequences in sporadic pediatric ependymomas. *Genes Chromosomes and Cancer*, 1996 17, 37-44.

[52] Ebert, C; von Haken, M; Meyer-Puttlitz, B; Wiestler, OD; Reifenberger, G; Pietsch, T; von Deimling, A. Molecular genetic analysis of ependymal tumors. NF2 mutations and chromosome 22q loss occur preferentially in intramedullary spinal ependymomas. *American Journal of Pathology*, 1999 155, 627-632.

[53] Buccoliero, AM; Castiglione, F; Rossi Degl'Innocenti, D; Sardi, I; Genitori, L; Taddei, GL. Merlin expression in pediatric anaplastic ependymomas real time PCR study. *Fetal and Pediatric Pathology*, 2010 29, 245-254.

[54] Mullins, KJ; Rubio, A; Myers, SP; Korones, DN; Pilcher, WH. Malignant ependymomas in a patient with Turcot's syndrome: case report and management guidelines. *Surgical Neurology*, 1998 49, 290-294.

[55] Metzger, AK; Sheffield, VC; Duyk, G; Daneshvar, L; Edwards, MS; Cogen, PH. Identification of a germ-line mutation in the p53 gene in a patient with an intracranial ependymoma. *Proceedings of the National Academy of Sciences of the United States of America*, 1991 88, 7825-7829.

[56] Nijssen, PC; Deprez, RH; Tijssen, CC; Hagemeijer, A; Arnoldus, EP; Teepen, JL; Holl, R; Niermeyer, MF. Familial anaplastic ependymoma: evidence of loss of chromosome 22 in tumour cells. *Journal of Neurology, Neurosurgery, and Psychiatry*, 1994 57, 1245-1248.

[57] Hulsebos, TJ; Oskam, NT; Bijleveld, EH; Westerveld, A; Hermsen, MA; van den Ouweland, AM; Hamel, BC; Tijssen, CC. Evidence for an ependymoma tumour suppressor gene in chromosome region 22pter-22q11.2. *British Journal of Cancer*, 1999 81, 1150-1154.

[58] Yokota, T; Tachizawa, T; Fukino, K; Teramoto, A; Kouno, J; Matsumoto, K; Emi, M. A family with spinal anaplastic ependymoma: evidence of loss of chromosome 22q in tumor. *Journal of Human Genetics*, 2003 48, 598-602.

[59] Dimopoulos, VG; Fountas, KN; Robinson, JS. Familial intracranial ependymomas. Report of three cases in a family and review of the literature. *Neurosurgical Focus*, 2006 20, E8.

[60] Yao, Y; Mack, SC; Taylor, MD. Molecular genetics of ependymoma. *Chinese Journal of Cancer*, 2011 30, 669-681.

[61] Taylor, MD; Poppleton, H; Fuller, C; Su, X; Liu, Y; Jensen, P; Magdaleno, S; Dalton, J; Calabrese, C; Board, J; Macdonald, T; Rutka, J; Guha, A; Gajjar, A; Curran, T; Gilbertson, RJ. Radialglia cells are candidate stem cells of ependymoma. *Cancer Cell*, 2005 8, 323-335.

[62] Palm, T; Figarella-Branger, D; Chapon, F; Lacroix, C; Gray, F; Scaravilli, F; Ellison, DW; Salmon, I; Vikkula, M; Godfraind, C. Expression profiling of ependymomas unravels localization and tumor grade-specific tumorigenesis. *Cancer*, 2009 115, 3955-3968.

[63] Johnson, RA; Wright, KD; Poppleton, H; Mohankumar, KM; Finkelstein, D; Pounds, SB; Rand, V; Leary, SE; White, E; Eden, C; Hogg, T; Northcott, P; Mack, S; Neale, G; Wang, YD; Coyle, B; Atkinson, J; DeWire, M; Kranenburg, TA; Gillespie, Y; Allen, JC; Merchant, T; Boop, FA; Sanford, RA; Gajjar, A; Ellison, DW; Taylor, MD; Grundy, RG; Gilbertson, RJ. Cross-species genomics matches driver mutations and cell compartments to model ependymoma. *Nature*, 2010 466, 632-636.

[64] Scheil, S; Brüderlein, S; Eicker, M; Herms, J; Herold-Mende, C; Steiner, HH; Barth, TF; Möller, P. Low frequency of chromosomal imbalances in anaplastic ependymomas as detected by comparative genomic hybridization. *Brain Pathology*, 2001 11, 133-143.

[65] Rousseau, A; Idbaih, A; Ducray, F; Crinière, E; Fèvre-Montange, M; Jouvet, A; Delattre, JY. Specific chromosomal imbalances as detected by array CGH in ependymomas in association with tumor location, histological subtype and grade. *Journal of Neurooncology*, 2010 97, 353-364.

[66] Hirose, Y; Aldape, K; Bollen, A; James, CD; Brat, D; Lamborn, K; Berger, M; Feuerstein, BG. Chromosomal abnormalities subdivide ependymal tumors into clinically relevant groups. *The American Journal of Pathology*, 2001 158, 1137-1143.

[67] Huang, B; Starostik, P; Schraut, H; Krauss, J; Sörensen, N; Roggendorf, W. Human ependymomas reveal frequent deletions on chromosomes 6 and 9. *Acta Neuropathologica*, 2003 106 357-362.

[68] Mendrzyk, F; Korshunov, A; Benner, A; Toedt, G; Pfister, S; Radlwimmer, B; Lichter, P. Identification of gains on 1q and epidermal growth factor receptor overexpression as independent prognostic markers in intracranial ependymoma. *Clinical Cancer Research*, 2006 12, 2070-2079.

[69] Hasselblatt, M. Ependymal tumors. *Recent Results Cancer Research*, 2009 171, 51-66.

[70] Ward, S; Harding, B; Wilkins, P; Harkness, W; Hayward, R; Darling, JL; Thomas, DG; Warr, T. Gain of 1q and loss of 22 are the most common changes detected by comparative genomic hybridisation in paediatric ependymoma. *Genes Chromosomes Cancer*, 2001 32, 59-66.

[71] Mack, SC; Taylor, MD. The genetic and epigenetic basis of ependymoma. *Childs Nervous System*, 2009 25, 1195-1201.

[72] Dyer, S; Prebble, E; Davison, V; Davies, P; Ramani, P; Ellison, D; Grundy, R. Genomic imbalances in pediatric intracranial ependymomas define clinically relevant groups. *American Journal of Pathology*, 2002 161, 2133-2141.

[73] Carter, M; Nicholson, J; Ross, F; Crolla, J; Allibone, R; Balaji, V; Perry, R; Walker, D; Gilbertson, R; Ellison, DW. Genetic abnormalities detected in ependymomas by comparative genomic hybridisation. *British Journal of Cancer*, 2002 86, 929-939.

[74] Pfister, S; Hartmann, C; Korshunov, A. Histology and molecular pathology of pediatric brain tumors. *Journal of Child Neurology*, 2009 24, 1375-1386.

[75] Korshunov, A; Witt, H; Hielscher, T; Benner, A; Remke, M; Ryzhova, M; Milde, T; Bender, S; Wittmann, A; Schöttler, A; Kulozik, AE; Witt, O; von Deimling, A; Lichter, P; Pfister, S. Molecular staging of intracranial ependymoma in children and adults. *Journal of Clinical Oncology*, 2010 28, 3182-3190.

[76] Puget, S; Grill, J; Valent, A; Bieche, I; Dantas-Barbosa, C; Kauffmann, A; Dessen, P; Lacroix, L; Geoerger, B; Job, B; Dirven, C; Varlet, P; Peyre, M; Dirks, PB; Sainte-Rose, C; Vassal, G. Candidate genes on chromosome 9q33-34 involved in the progression of childhood ependymomas. *Journal of Clinical Oncology*, 2009 27, 1884-1892.

[77] Zhang, XM; Dormady, SP; Chaung W; Basch, RS. mVH1, a dual-specificity phosphatase whose expression is cell cycle regulated. *Mammalian Genome*, 2000 11, 1154-1156.

[78] Sharda, PR; Bonham, CA; Mucaki, EJ; Butt, Z; Vacratsis, PO. The dual-specificity phosphatase hYVH1 interacts with Hsp70 and prevents heat-shock-induced cell death. *The Biochemical Journal*, 2009 418, 391-401.

[79] Almeida, A; Zhu, XX; Vogt, N; Tyagi, R; Muleris, M; Dutrillaux, AM; Dutrillaux, B; Ross, D; Malfoy, B; Hanash, S. GAC1, a new member of the leucine-rich repeat superfamily on chromosome band 1q32.1, is amplified and overexpressed in malignant gliomas. *Oncogene*, 1998 16, 2997-3002.

[80] Suarez-Merino, B; Hubank, M; Revesz, T; Harkness, W; Hayward, R; Thompson, D; Darling, JL; Thomas, DG; Warr, TJ. Microarray analysis of pediatric ependymoma identifies a cluster of 112 candidate genes including four transcripts at 22q12.1-q13.3. *Neuro-Oncology*, 2005 7, 20-31.

[81] Karakoula, K; Suarez-Merino, B; Ward, S; Phipps, KP; Harkness, W; Hayward, R; Thompson, D; Jacques, TS; Harding, B; Beck, J; Thomas, DG; Warr, TJ. Real-time quantitative PCR analysis of pediatric ependymomas identifies novel candidate genes including TPR at 1q25 and CHIBBY at 22q12-q13. *Genes Chromosomes Cancer*, 2008 47, 1005-1022.

[82] Rand, V; Prebble, E; Ridley, L; Howard, M; Wei, W; Brundler, MA; Fee, BE; Riggins, GJ; Coyle, B; Grundy, RG. Children's Cancer and Leukaemia Group Biological Studies Committee. Investigation of chromosome 1q reveals differential expression of members of the S100 family in clinical subgroups of intracranial paediatric ependymoma. *British Journal of Cancer*, 2008 99, 1136-1143.

[83] Hirai, M; Yoshida, S; Kashiwagi, H; Kawamura, T; Ishikawa, T; Kaneko, M; Ohkawa, H; Nakagawara, A; Miwa, M; Uchida, K. 1q23 gain is associated with progressive neuroblastoma resistant to aggressive treatment. *Genes Chromosomes Cancer*, 1999 25, 261-269.

[84] Hing, S; Lu, YJ; Summersgill, B; King-Underwood, L; Nicholson, J; Grundy, P; Grundy, R; Gessler, M; Shipley, J; Pritchard-Jones, K. Gain of 1q is associated with

adverse outcome in favorable histology Wilms' tumors. *American Journal of Pathology*, 2001 158, 393-398.

[85] Ozaki, T; Paulussen, M; Poremba, C; Brinkschmidt, C; Rerin, J; Ahrens, S; Hoffmann, C; Hillmann, A; Wai, D; Schaefer, KL; Boecker, W; Juergens, H; Winkelmann, W; Dockhorn-Dworniczak, B. Genetic imbalances revealed by comparative genomic hybridization in Ewing tumors. *Genes Chromosomes Cancer*, 2001 32, 164-171.

[86] Schneider, D; Monoranu, CM; Huang, B; Rutkowski, S; Gerber, NU; Krauss, J; Puppe, B; Roggendorf, W. Pediatric supratentorial ependymomas show more frequent deletions on chromosome 9 than infratentorial ependymomas: a microsatellite analysis. *Cancer Genetics and Cytogenetics*, 2009 191, 90-96.

[87] Monoranu, CM; Huang, B; Zangen, IL; Rutkowski, S; Vince, GH; Gerber, NU; Puppe, B; Roggendorf, W. Correlation between 6q25.3 deletion status and survival in pediatric intracranial ependymomas. *Cancer Genetics and Cytogenetics*, 2008 182, 18-26.

[88] Bortolotto, S; Chiadò-Piat, L; Cavalla, P; Bosone, I; Mauro, A; Schiffer, D. CDKN2A/p16 in ependymomas. *Journal of Neurooncology*, 2001 54, 9-13.

[89] Nishiyama, H; Takahashi, T; Kakehi, Y; Habuchi, T; Knowles, MA. Homozygous deletion at the 9q32-33 candidate tumor suppressor locus in primary human bladder cancer. *Genes, Chromosomes and Cancer*, 1999 26, 171-175.

[90] Beetz, C; Brodoehl, S; Patt, S; Kalff, R; Deufel, T. Low expression but infrequent genomic loss of the putative tumour suppressor DBCCR1 in astrocytoma. *Oncology Reports*, 2005 13, 335-340.

[91] Milde, T; Pfister, S; Korshunov, A; Deubzer, HE; Oehme, I; Ernst, A; Starzinski-Powitz, A; Seitz, A; Lichter, P; von Deimling, A; Witt, O. Stepwise accumulation of distinct genomic aberrations in a patient with progressively metastasizing ependymoma. *Genes, Chromosomes and Cancer*, 2009 48, 229-238.

[92] Bharti, S; Handrow-Metzmacher, H; Zickenheiner, S; Zeitvogel, A; Baumann, R; Starzinski-Powitz, A. Novel membrane protein shrew-1 targets to cadherin-mediated junctions in polarized epithelial cells. *Molecular Biology of the Cell*, 2004 15, 397-406.

[93] Mack, SC; Witt, H; Piro, RM; Gu, L; Zuyderduyn, S; Stütz, AM; Wang, X; Gallo, M; Garzia, L; Zayne, K; Zhang, X; Ramaswamy, V; Jäger, N; Jones, DT; Sill, M; Pugh, TJ; Ryzhova, M; Wani, KM; Shih, DJ; Head, R; Remke, M; Bailey, SD; Zichner, T; Faria, CC; Barszczyk, M; Stark, S; Seker-Cin, H; Hutter, S; Johann, P; Bender, S; Hovestadt, V; Tzaridis, T; Dubuc, AM; Northcott, PA; Peacock, J; Bertrand, KC; Agnihotri, S; Cavalli, FM; Clarke, I; Nethery-Brokx, K; Creasy, CL; Verma, SK; Koster, J; Wu, X; Yao, Y; Milde, T; Sin-Chan, P; Zuccaro, J; Lau, L; Pereira, S; Castelo-Branco, P; Hirst, M; Marra, MA; Roberts, SS; Fults, D; Massimi, L; Cho, YJ; Van Meter, T; Grajkowska, W; Lach, B; Kulozik, AE; von Deimling, A; Witt, O; Scherer, SW; Fan, X; Muraszko, KM; Kool, M; Pomeroy, SL; Gupta, N; Phillips, J; Huang, A; Tabori, U; Hawkins, C; Malkin, D; Kongkham, PN; Weiss, WA; Jabado, N; Rutka, JT; Bouffet, E; Korbel, JO; Lupien, M; Aldape, KD; Bader, GD; Eils, R; Lichter, P; Dirks, PB; Pfister, SM; Korshunov, A; Taylor, MD. Epigenomic alterations define lethal CIMP-positive ependymomas of infancy. *Nature*, 2014 506, 445-450.

[94] McDonald, JM; Dunlap, S; Cogdell, D; Dunmire, V; Wei, Q; Starzinski-Powitz, A; Sawaya, R; Bruner, J; Fuller, GN; Aldape, K; Zhang, W. The SHREW1 gene,

frequently deleted in oligodendrogliomas, functions to inhibit cell adhesion and migration. *Cancer Biology and Therapy*, 2006 5, 300-304.

[95] Schreiner, A; Ruonala, M; Jakob, V; Suthaus, J; Boles, E; Wouters, F; Starzinski-Powitz, A. Junction protein shrew-1 influences cell invasion and interacts with invasion-promoting protein CD147. *Molecular Biology of the Cell*, 2007 18, 1272-1281.

[96] Rogers, HA; Kilday, JP; Mayne, C; Ward, J; Adamowicz-Brice, M; Schwalbe, EC; Clifford, SC; Coyle, B; Grundy, RG. Supratentorial and spinal pediatric ependymomas display a hypermethylated phenotype, which includes the loss of tumor suppressor genes involved in the control of cell growth and death. *Acta Neuropathologica*, 2012 123, 711-725.

[97] Toyota, M; Ahuja, N; Ohe-Toyota, M; Herman, JG; Baylin, SB; Issa, JP. CpG island methylator phenotype in colorectal cancer. *Proceedings of the National Academy of Sciences of the United States of America*, 1999 96, 8681-8686.

[98] Noushmehr, H; Weisenberger, DJ; Diefes, K; Phillips, HS; Pujara, K; Berman, BP; Pan, F; Pelloski, CE; Sulman, EP; Bhat, KP; Verhaak, RG; Hoadley, KA; Hayes, DN; Perou, CM; Schmidt, HK; Ding, L; Wilson, RK; Van Den Berg, D; Shen, H; Bengtsson, H; Neuvial, P; Cope, LM; Buckley, J; Herman, JG; Baylin, SB; Laird, PW; Aldape, K; Cancer Genome Atlas Research Network. Identification of a CpG island methylator phenotype that defines a distinct subgroup of glioma. *Cancer Cell,* 2010 17, 510-522.

[99] Mack, SC; Witt, H; Wang, X; Milde, T; Yao, Y; Bertrand, KC; Korshunov, A; Pfister, SM; Taylor, MD. Emerging insights into the ependymoma epigenome. *Brain Pathology*, 2013 23, 206-209.

[100] Fu, HY; Wu, DS; Zhou, HR; Shen, JZ. CpG island methylator phenotype and its relationship with prognosis in adult acute leukemia patients. *Hematology*, 2014 19, 329-337.

[101] Hamilton, DW; Lusher, ME; Lindsey, JC; Ellison, DW; Clifford, SC. Epigenetic inactivation of the RASSF1A tumour suppressor gene in ependymoma. *Cancer Letters,* 2005 227, 75-81.

[102] Donninger, H; Vos, MD; Clark, GJ. The RASSF1A tumor suppressor. *Journal of Cell Science*, 2007 120, 3163-3172.

[103] Waha, A; Koch, A; Hartmann, W; Mack, H; Schramm, J; Sörensen, N; Berthold, F; Wiestler, OD; Pietsch, T; Waha, A. Analysis of HIC-1 methylation and transcription in human ependymomas. *International Journal of Cancer*, 2004 110, 542-549.

[104] Rousseau, E; Ruchoux, MM; Scaravilli, F; Chapon, F; Vinchon, M; De Smet, C; Godfraind, C; Vikkula, M. CDKN2A, CDKN2B and p14ARF are frequently and differentially methylated in ependymal tumours. *Neuropathology and Applied Neurobiology*, 2003 29, 574-583.

[105] Buccoliero, AM; Castiglione, F; Rossi Degl'Innocenti, D; Paglierani, M; Maio, V; Gheri, CF; Garbini, F; Moncini, D; Taddei, A; Sardi, I; Sanzo, M; Giordano, F; Mussa, F; Genitori, L; Taddei, GL. O6-Methylguanine-DNA-methyltransferase in recurring anaplastic ependymomas: PCR and immunohistochemistry. *Journal of Chemotherapy*, 2008 20, 263-268.

[106] Danielsson, A; Nemes, S; Tisell, M; Lannering, B; Nordborg, C; Sabel, M; Carén, H. MethPed: a DNA methylation classifier tool for the identification of pediatric brain tumor subtypes. *Clinical Epigenetics*, 2015 7, 62.
[107] Korshunov, A; Neben, K; Wrobel, G; Tews, B; Benner, A; Hahn, M; Golanov, A; Lichter, P. Gene expression patterns in ependymomas correlate with tumor location, grade, and patient age. *The American Journal of Pathology*, 2003 163, 1721-1727.
[108] Lukashova-v Zangen, I; Kneitz, S; Monoranu, CM; Rutkowski, S; Hinkes, B; Vince, GH; Huang, B; Roggendorf, W. Ependymoma gene expression profiles associated with histological subtype, proliferation, and patient survival. *Acta Neuropathologica*, 2007 113, 325-337.
[109] Witt, H; Mack, SC; Ryzhova, M; Bender, S; Sill, M; Isserlin, R; Benner, A; Hielscher, T; Milde, T; Remke, M; Jones, DT; Northcott, PA; Garzia, L; Bertrand, KC; Wittmann, A; Yao, Y; Roberts, SS; Massimi, L; Van Meter, T; Weiss, WA; Gupta, N; Grajkowska, W; Lach, B; Cho, YJ; von Deimling, A; Kulozik, AE; Witt, O; Bader, GD; Hawkins, CE; Tabori, U; Guha; A; Rutka, JT; Lichter, P; Korshunov, A; Taylor, MD; Pfister, SM. Delineation of two clinically and molecularly distinct subgroups of posterior fossa ependymoma. *Cancer Cell*, 2011 20,143-157.
[110] Wani, K; Armstrong, TS; Vera-Bolanos, E; Raghunathan, A; Ellison, D; Gilbertson, R; Vaillant, B; Goldman, S; Packer, RJ; Fouladi, M; Pollack, I; Mikkelsen, T; Prados, M; Omuro, A; Soffietti, R; Ledoux, A; Wilson, C; Long, L; Gilbert, MR; Aldape, K; Collaborative Ependymoma Research Network. A prognostic gene expression signature in infratentorial ependymoma. *Acta Neuropathologica*, 2012 123, 727-738.
[111] Hirahara, F; Yamanaka, M; Miyagia, E; Nakazawa, T; Gorai, I; Minaguchi, H; Kakei, M; Yamamoto, M; Kitamura, H. Pure ovarian ependymoma: report of a case treated with surgery, chemotherapy, irradiation and hyperthermotherapy. *European Journal of Obstetrics, Gynecology, and Reproductive Biology*, 1997 75, 221-223.
[112] Neumann, DP; Scholl, RJ; Kellet, HM; Simon, RH. Magnetic resonance imaging of a mediastinal ependymoma. *Connecticut Medicine*, 1998 62, 527-530.
[113] Aktuğ, T; Hakgüder, G; Sarioğlu, S; Akgür, FM; Olguner, M; Pabuçcuoğlu, U. Sacrococcygeal extraspinal ependymomas: the role of coccygectomy. *Journal of Pediatric Surgery*, 2000 35, 515-518.
[114] Zacharoulis, S; Levy, A; Chi, SN; Gardner, S; Rosenblum, M; Miller, DC; Dunkel, I; Diez, B; Sposto, R; Ji, L; Asgharzadeh, S; Hukin, J; Belasco, J; Dubowy, R; Kellie, S; Termuhlen, A; Finlay, J. Outcome for young children newly diagnosed with ependymoma, treated with intensive induction chemotherapy followed by myeloablative chemotherapy and autologous stem cell rescue. *Pediatric Blood and Cancer*, 2007 49, 34-40.
[115] Paulino, AC. Radiotherapeutic management of intracranial ependymoma. *Pediatric Hematology and Oncology*. 2002 19, 295-308.
[116] Perilongo, G; Massimino, M; Sotti, G; Belfontali, T; Masiero, L; Rigobello, L; Garrè, L; Carli, M; Lombardi, F; Solero, C; Sainati, L; Canale, V; del Prever, AB; Giangaspero, F; Andreussi, L; Mazza, C; Madon, E. Analyses of prognostic factors in a retrospective review of 92 children with ependymoma: Italian Pediatric Neuro-oncology Group. *Medical and Pediatric Oncology*, 1997 29, 79-85.

[117] Massimino, M; Gandola, L; Giangaspero, F; Sandri, A; Valagussa, P; Perilongo, G; Garrè, ML; Ricardi, U; Forni, M; Genitori, L; Scarzello, G; Spreafico, F; Barra, S; Mascarin, M; Pollo, B; Gardiman, M; Cama, A; Navarria, P; Brisigotti, M; Collini, P; Balter, R; Fidani, P; Stefanelli, M; Burnelli, R; Potepan, P; Podda, M; Sotti, G; Madon, E; AIEOP Pediatric Neuro-Oncology Group. Hyperfractionated radiotherapy and chemotherapy for childhood ependymoma: final results of the first prospective AIEOP (Associazione Italiana di Ematologia-Oncologia Pediatrica) study. *International Journal of Radiation Oncology, Biology, Physics*, 2004 58, 1336-1345.

[118] Rickert, CH; Paulus, W. Prognosis-related histomorphological and immunohistochemical markers in central nervous system tumors of childhood and adolescence. *Acta Neuropathologica*, 2005 109, 69-92.

[119] Korshunov, A; Golanov, A; Sycheva, R; Timirgaz, V. The histologic grade is a main prognostic factor for patients with intracranial ependymomas treated in the microneurosurgical era: an analysis of 258 patients. *Cancer*, 2004 100, 1230-1237.

[120] Rodríguez, D; Cheung, MC; Housri, N; Quinones-Hinojosa, A; Camphausen, K; Koniaris, LG. Outcomes of malignant CNS ependymomas: an examination of 2408 cases through the Surveillance, Epidemiology, and End Results (SEER) database (1973-2005). *The Journal of Surgical Research*, 2009 156, 340-351.

[121] Ellison, DW; Kocak, M; Figarella-Branger, D; Felice, G; Catherine, G; Pietsch, T; Frappaz, D; Massimino, M; Grill, J; Boyett, JM; Grundy, RG. Histopathological grading of pediatric ependymoma: reproducibility and clinical relevance in European trial cohorts. *Journal of Negative Results in Biomedicine,* 2011 10, 7.

[122] Armstrong, TS; Vera-Bolanos, E; Bekele, BN; Aldape, K; Gilbert, MR. Adult ependymal tumors: prognosis and the M. D. Anderson Cancer Center experience. *Neuro-Oncology*, 2010 12, 862-870.

[123] Messahel, B; Ashley, S; Saran, F; Ellison, D; Ironside, J; Phipps, K; Cox, T; Chong, WK; Robinson, K; Picton, S; Pinkerton, CR; Mallucci, C; Macarthur, D; Jaspan, T; Michalski, A; Grundy, RG; Children's Cancer Leukaemia Group Brain Tumour Committee. Relapsed intracranial ependymoma in children in the UK: patterns of relapse, survival and therapeutic outcome. *European Journal of Cancer*, 2009 45, 1815-1823.

[124] Andreiuolo, F; Puget, S; Peyre, M; Dantas-Barbosa, C; Boddaert, N; Philippe, C; Mauguen, A; Grill, J; Varlet, P. Neuronal differentiation distinguishes supratentorial and infratentorial childhood ependymomas. *Neuro-Oncology*, 2010 12, 1126-1134.

[125] Kilday, JP; Mitra, B; Domerg, C; Ward, J; Andreiuolo, F; Osteso-Ibanez, T; Mauguen, A; Varlet, P; Le Deley, MC; Lowe, J; Ellison, DW; Gilbertson, RJ; Coyle, B; Grill, J; Grundy, RG. Copy number gain of 1q25 predicts poor progression-free survival for pediatric intracranial ependymomas and enables patient risk stratification: a prospective European clinical trial cohort analysis on behalf of the Children's Cancer Leukaemia Group (CCLG), Societè Francaise d'Oncologie Pediatrique (SFOP), and International Society for Pediatric Oncology (SIOP). *Clinical Cancer Research*, 2012 18, 2001-2011.

[126] Godfraind, C; Kaczmarska, JM; Kocak, M; Dalton, J; Wright, KD; Sanford, RA; Boop, FA; Gajjar, A; Merchant, TE; Ellison, DW. Distinct disease-risk groups in pediatric

supratentorial and posterior fossa ependymomas. *Acta Neuropathologica*, 2012 124, 247-257.

[127] Costa, FF; Bischof, JM; Vanin, EF; Lulla, RR; Wang, M; Sredni, ST; Rajaram, V; Bonaldo Mde, F; Wang, D; Goldman, S; Tomita, T; Soares, MB. Identification of microRNAs as potential prognostic markers in ependymoma. *PLoSOne*, 2011 6, e25114.

[128] Bruce, NJ. Ependymoma treatment and management. *Drugs, Diseases and Procedures*, April 14, 2015. http://emedicine.medscape.com/article/277621-treatment.

[129] Cage, TA; Clark, AJ; Aranda, D; Gupta, N; Sun, PP; Parsa, AT; Auguste, KI. A systematic review of treatment outcomes in pediatric patients with intracranial ependymomas. *Journal of Neurosurgery Pediatrics*, 2013 11, 673-681.

[130] Chen, P; Sui, M; Ye, J; Wan, Z; Chen, F; Luo, C. An integrative analysis of treatment, outcomes and prognostic factors for primary spinal anaplastic ependymomas. *Journal of Clinical Neuroscience*, 2015 22, 976-980.

[131] Komori, K; Yanagisawa, R; Miyairi, Y; Sakashita, K; Shiohara, M; Fujihara, I; Morita, D; Nakamura, T; Ogiso, Y; Sano, K; Shirahata, M; Fukuoka, K; Ichimura, K; Shigeta, H. Temozolomide treatment for pediatric refractory anaplastic ependymoma with low MGMT protein expression. *Pediatric Blood and Cancer*, 2015. [Epub ahead of print]

[132] Hirono, S; Iwadate, Y; Kambe, M; Hiwasa, T; Takiguchi, M; Nakatani, Y; Saeki, N. Role of Evaluating MGMT Status and 1p36 deletion in radiosurgery-induced anaplastic ependymoma that rapidly and completely resolved by temozolomide alone: Case Report and Review of the Literature. *Journal of Neurological Surgery Reports*, 2015 76, e43-47.

[133] Stupp, R; Mason, WP; van den Bent, MJ; Weller, M; Fisher, B; Taphoorn, MJ; Belanger, K; Brandes, AA; Marosi, C; Bogdahn, U; Curschmann, J; Janzer, RC; Ludwin, SK; European Organisation for Research and Treatment of Cancer Brain Tumor and Radiotherapy Groups; National Cancer Institute of Canada Clinical Trials Group. Radiotherapy plus concomitant and adjuvant temozolomide for glioblastoma. *The New England Journal of Medicine*, 2005 352, 987-996.

[134] Rudà, R; Bosa, C; Magistrello, M; Franchino, F; Pellerino, A; Fiano, V; Trevisan, M; Cassoni, P; Soffietti, R. Temozolomide as salvage treatment for recurrent intracranial ependymomas of the adult: a retrospective study. *Neuro-Oncology*, 2015. [Epub ahead of print]

[135] Sandberg, DI; Rytting, M; Zaky, W; Kerr, M; Ketonen, L; Kundu, U; Moore, BD; Yang, G; Hou, P; Sitton, C; Cooper, LJ; Gopalakrishnan, V; Lee, DA; Thall, PF; Khatua, S. Methotrexate administration directly into the fourth ventricle in children with malignant fourth ventricular brain tumors: a pilot clinical trial. *Journal of Neurooncology*, 2015 125, 133-141.

[136] Eaton, BR; Chowdhry, V; Weaver, K; Liu, L; Ebb, D; MacDonald, SM; Tarbell, NJ; Yock, TI. Use of proton therapy for re-irradiation in pediatric intracranial ependymoma. *Radiotherapy and Oncology*, 2015 116, 301-308.

[137] Barszczyk, M; Buczkowicz, P; Castelo-Branco, P; Mack, SC; Ramaswamy, V; Mangerel, J; Agnihotri, S; Remke, M; Golbourn, B; Pajovic, S; Elizabeth, C; Yu, M; Luu, B; Morrison, A; Adamski, J; Nethery-Brokx, K; Li XN; Van Meter, T; Dirks PB; Rutka, JT; Taylor, MD; Tabori, U; Hawkins, C. Telomerase inhibition abolishes the

tumorigenicity of pediatric ependymoma tumor-initiating cells. *Acta Neuropathologica*, 2014 128, 863-877.

[138] Rahman, R; Osteso-Ibanez, T; Hirst, RA; Levesley, J; Kilday, JP; Quinn, S; Peet, A; O'Callaghan, C; Coyle, B; Grundy, RG. Histone deacetylase inhibition attenuates cell growth with associated telomerase inhibition in high-grade childhood brain tumor cells. *Molecular Cancer Therapeutics*, 2010 9, 2568-2581.

[139] Milde, T; Kleber, S; Korshunov, A; Witt, H; Hielscher, T; Koch, P; Kopp, HG; Jugold, M; Deubzer, HE; Oehme, I; Lodrini, M; Gröne, HJ; Benner, A; Brüstle, O; Gilbertson, RJ; von Deimling, A; Kulozik, AE; Pfister, SM; Martin-Villalba, A; Witt, O. A novel human high-risk ependymoma stem cell model reveals the differentiation-inducing potential of the histone deacetylase inhibitor Vorinostat. *Acta Neuropathologica*, 2011 122, 637-650.

In: Ependymomas
Editor: Raquel Fowler

ISBN: 978-1-63484-405-5

Chapter 4

Intramedullary and Myxopapillary Ependymomas: An Evidence-Based Approach

Nicandro Figueiredo, MD, MSc, PhD[1,*]
and Sergio Castelo B. F. Santana, MD[2]

[1]Spinal Neurosurgeon, Medcare Orthopaedics and Spine Hospital, Dubai, UAE; Honorary Fellow, Department of Neurological Surgery, University of Wisconsin, Madison, US (2011-2015); Professor, Medical School, Federal University of Mato Grosso and University of Cuiaba, Cuiaba, MT, Brazil

[2]Neuroradiologist, CEDIC; Professor of Radiology, Medical School, University of Cuiaba, Cuiaba, MT, Brazil

Abstract

Background: Intraspinal ependymomas (ISE) constitute approximately 60% of all intradural spinal tumors; around 50% are **intramedullary ependymoma (IME)** and the remaining **myxopapillary ependymoma (MPE)**.

Methods: This chapter contains a contemporary **review** of the **literature** and an **evidence-based systematic review** about **ISE**. A published case series of the **University of Wisconsin Hospital (UWH),** of patients operated upon for **ISE**, was also presented to illustrate this manuscript. All this information was properly discussed in order to propose guidelines for the management of patients with ISE.

Results: This chapter was written based on the review of many relevant and updated scientific sources, including the author's **evidence-based systematic review** about **ISE,** based on 27 papers (1,211 patients). A review of series regarding **IME** was based on 4 papers (143 patients). The overall recurrence/progression rate was 3.63%. The highest incidence of recurrence occurred in patients submitted to subtotal resection (STR) alone

[*] Corresponding author: Dr. Nicandro Figueiredo, Spinal Neurosurgeon, Medcare Orthopaedics & Spine Hospital (MOSH); Sheikh Zayed Road; exit 47; P.O. Box 215565 Dubai, UAE, Office: +971 4 3768414; E-mail: nicandro2@yahoo.com.

(5.26%), followed by GTR alone (3.37%). The review regarding **MPE** was based on 5 papers (199 patients). The overall recurrence/progression rate was 24.12%. Gross-total resection (GTR) alone resulted in 15.21% of recurrence, while GTR plus radiotherapy (XRT) reduced the recurrence rate to 5.26%. The published **UWH case series** of 38 patients was also described. Nineteen patients were operated for **IME**. GTR was achieved in 11, being 4 *en bloc* GTR, 6 piecemeal, not specified in 1 case, and all remained disease-free. STR was accomplished in 6 patients, 3 were living with stable disease; 2 with progression of the neoplasm, and 1 died after the tumor progression. Partial removal was performed in 2 patients, they were submitted to XRT, 1 deceased, and another was living with stable tumor. Eleven were disease-free, and 8 had tumor recurrence, progression and/or stable disease. Nineteen patients had **MPE.** GTR was achieved in 14, seven *en bloc* GTR, all remained disease-free, 7 piecemeal GTR, and 2 cases had tumor recurrence. STR was accomplished in 2, they were submitted to XRT, and they were living with stable disease. Partial resection was performed in 2, they were re-operated and submitted to XRT, and were living with the neoplasm. Biopsy was performed in 1 patient. Thirteen patients remained disease-free and 6 had tumor recurrence, progression and/or stable disease.

Conclusions: This manuscript was based on **level IV of medical evidence (recommendation grade C)** supporting that **early diagnosis and better preoperative neurological status** can improve the postoperative neurological **outcome** in patients treated with **ISE;** supporting the **role of GTR**; supporting **postoperative XRT** to reduce the recurrence/progression of the tumor in patients with **ISE submitted to incomplete resection**; and also supporting the use of **routine postoperative XRT** to potentially reduce the recurrence/progression of the tumor in patients **operated for MPE**, even after GTR. Intraspinal ependymoma is not as "benign" as proposed by its histology, but has a high potential of recurrence and/or progression. In this chapter we describe the clinical symptoms of intramedullary tumors and their neuroradiological features, provide a description of modern surgical techniques, and discuss the postoperative results and outcomes on the basis of UWH series and the evidence-based systematic review of the literature.

Keywords: intraspinal ependymomas, spinal cord ependymoma, myxopapillary ependymoma, ependymoma, intradural spinal tumor, spinal cord tumor

General concepts regarding evidence-based medicine for spine care

Evidence-based medicine (EBM) is the conscientious, explicit and judicious use of current best evidence in making decisions about the care of individual patients. The use of mathematical estimates of the risk of benefit and harm, derived from high-quality research on population samples, to inform clinical decision-making in the diagnosis, investigation or management of individual patients. EBM seeks to assess the strength of the evidence of risks and benefits of treatments (including lack of treatment) and diagnostic tests. This helps clinicians predict whether a treatment will do more good than harm [19, 50].

The Evidence-Based Clinical Guidelines Committee for Multidisciplinary Spine Care of the North American Spine Society (NASS) has adopted standardized levels of evidence and grades of recommendation to assist practitioners in easily understanding the strength of the evidence, and to give recommendations within the guidelines [22].

The **levels of evidence** range from Level I (high quality randomized controlled trial) to Level V (expert consensus). **Grades of recommendation** indicate the strength of the recommendations made in the guideline based on the quality of the literature [22].

- **NASS assessment of medical evidence**
    - **Level I**
        - Well-designed randomized controlled clinical trials (RCT)
        - Systematic review (SR) of well-designed RCT
    - **Level II**
        - Prospective comparative studies
        - SR of level II studies
    - **Level III**
        - Case control studies
        - Retrospective comparative studies
        - SR of level III studies
    - **Level IV**
        - Case series
    - **Level V**
        - Expert opinion

Guideline recommendations are written utilizing a standard language that indicates the strength of the recommendation. "A" recommendations indicate a test or intervention is "recommended"; "B" recommendations "suggest" a test or intervention; and "C" recommendations indicate a test or intervention "may be considered" or "is an option." "I" or "Insufficient Evidence" statements clearly indicate that "there is insufficient evidence to make a recommendation for or against" a test or intervention. Work group consensus statements clearly state that "in the absence of reliable evidence, it is the work group's opinion that" a test or intervention may be appropriate or not [22].

- **NASS strategy for recommendation grading**
    - **Grade A**
        - Good evidence (recommended)
            - 2 or more Level I studies with consistent findings
    - **Grade B**
        - Fair evidence (suggested)
            - Single Level I study or multiple level II or III with consistent findings
    - **Grade C**
        - Poor evidence (option)
            - Single Level II study or multiple level IV or V studies
    - **Grade I**
        - Insufficient evidence
            - Single Level III, IV or V studies of equivalent strength with conflicting findings/conclusions.

Intraspinal Ependymomas

Introduction

Intramedullary tumors are relatively rare, accounting for only 5 to 10% of all spinal tumors [5, 34, 35]. In adults, the intramedullary tumors comprise about one third of all intradural neoplasms, being about 45% ependymoma, 40% astrocytoma (oligodendroglioma, ganglioglioma, neurocytoma, and subependymoma), 5% hemangioblastoma and 10% miscellaneous (metastatic tumor, inclusion tumor, inflammation and vascular condition) [42].

A minority of intramedullary tumors is associated with genetic diseases such as von-Hippel-Lindau disease (VHL), causing hemangioblastomas and neurofibromatosis type 2 (NF-2) associated with ependymomas or astrocytomas. Intramedullary tumors are observed in 19% of patients with NF-2 and 20% of those with VHL. In neurofibromatosis type 1 (NF-1), intramedullary tumors are rare. So far, only astrocytomas have been encountered in NF-1 [65].

About 3% of CNS astrocytomas arise within the spinal cord, and are most prevalent in the first three decades of life. They are the most common pediatric intramedullary spinal cord tumor, comprising about 90% of intramedullary tumors in patients under 10 years of age and about 60% of adolescent intramedullary neoplasm. By about 30 years of age ependymomas become slightly more common than astrocytomas and increasingly predominate in the middle decades of life. After the sixth decade of life, astrocytomas and ependymomas are encountered with about equal frequency [30].

Ependymomas constitute 3% to 6% of all CNS tumors, 15% of all intraspinal tumors, and approximately 60% of all intramedullary tumors. They occur throughout life, but are most common in the middle adult years [7]. Spinal ependymomas are usually well circumscribed arising from ependymal cells lining the central canal or its remnants and from the cells of the ventriculus terminalis in the filum terminale. Hemorrhage and cystic degeneration are common [67]. Ependymomas are more common in the spinal cord than in intracranial regions across all age groups, being distributed like this: 36.2% in the spine, 22.2% infratentorial, and 11.8% in the supratentorial region, occurring more often in males (56.9%) [37].

Intramedullary ependymomas are the most common spinal cord tumors in adults. They occur throughout life but are most common in the middle adult years and equally affect men and women. Approximately 65% of patients will have associated syrinx, particularly when the tumor occupies a cervical or cervicothoracic location. There are a number of histologic subtypes, but the most common is the cellular ependymoma. These tumors are usually well circumscribed and do not infiltrate into the adjacent spinal cord, as astrocytomas do [34]. Almost all ependymomas are benign, grade II by the World Health Organization (WHO) classification, and only a few are anaplastic, classified as grade III [30].

Myxopapillary ependymomas of the filum terminale represent approximately 15% of intradural extramedullary tumors. They typically occur in adults and are the most common tumors to arise in the filum terminale. These tumors are benign, and their classic appearance is a papillary arrangement of cuboid or columnar epithelial cells with rich mucin content. Although these tumors arise from the filum terminale, they can secondarily involve the nerve roots of the cauda equina. They can also seed the spinal fluid compartment with "drop metastases", which necessitates adjuvant treatment [41, 49]. MPE is characterized by biphasic features composed of hypocellular myxoid regions intermixed with hypercellular papillary areas. These tumors usually grow slowly, but they can become large and can seed the subarachnoid space intracranially [2, 29]. Myxopapillary ependymomas are classified as grade I, by the WHO classification [30].

Table 1. Summary of the patients with intramedullary ependymomas from the University of Wisconsin Hospital series

INTRAMEDULLARY EPENDYMOMA		
IME	**Number (N)**	**Percentage (%)**
Number of patients	19	100%
Grade II – ependymoma	15	78.94%
Grade III – anaplastic ependymoma	4	21.05%
Non-specified or missing	0	
Location in the spine		
Number of regions affected in the spine	29	100%
Cervico-medullary	5	17.24%
Cervical	5	17.24%
Thoracic	10	34.48%
Lumbar (lumbosacral/cauda equina/terminal filum's region)	7	24.13%
Sacral	2	6.89%
Multiple locations and/or metastasis	6	
Gender		
Male	8	42.10%
Female	11	57.89%
Coexisting neoplastic condition		
CNS neoplasms	4	21.05%
Other neoplasms	1	5.26%
Neurofibromatosis type I (NF I)	2	10.52%
Neurofibromatosis type II (NF II)	2	10.52%
Other relevant spinal disease	6	31.57%
Age		
Mean age	40.95 years	
Range	14 to 84.41 years	
Clinical scenario		
Axial pain	17	89.47%
Radicular and/or referred pain	10	52.63%
Motor deficit	4	21.05%
Sensory deficit	7	36.84%
Coordination and/or balance	1	5.26%
Gait difficult	3	15.78%
Urinary disturbance	2	10.52%
Rectal disturbance	2	10.52%
Sexual dysfunction	0	0

Table 1. (Continued)

INTRAMEDULLARY EPENDYMOMA				
IME	**Number (N)**	**Percentage (%)**		
Spinal deformity	1	5.26%		
Mean duration of symptoms (before the 1st surgery)	12.93 months			
Diagnostic testing				
Pre-operative MRI	19	100%		
Postoperative MRI	19	100%		
Eletroneuromiography	3	15.78%		
Treatment of the IME				
Spinal surgery approach				
Patients operated for IME	19			
Number of surgical procedures to remove the tumor	23	100%		
Posterior or posterolateral approach	23	100%		
Laminectomy	17	73.9%		
Laminoplasty	6	26.1%		
Posterolateral fusion	4	15.38%		
Anterior or anterolateral approach	0	0		
Combined approach (front and back)	0	0		
Postoperative neurological result (last surgery)				
Unchanged	13	68.42%		
Improved	3	15.78%		
Deteriorated	3	15.78%		
McCormick functional grade (last surgery)	I	II	III	IV
Before surgery	14	3	2	0
Immediate after surgery	13	4	2	0
3 months after surgery	13	4	2	0
1 year after surgery	13	4	2	0
Latest follow-up (from the last surgery)	12	4	2	1
Mean follow-up (from the last surgery)	31.06 months			
Radiation therapy for IME				
Patients submitted to XRT	7	36.8%		
Complication related to the XRT	2	18.18%		
Chemotherapy for IME				
Patients submitted to CHT	1	5.26%		
Number of CHT	2	100%		
Systemic chemotherapy	2	100%		
Intrathecal chemotherapy	0	0		
Postoperative mortality (period)				
Short term (<1 month)				
Intraoperative	0	0		
<1 month	0	0		
Medium and long term	2	100%		
Mean death period	33 months			
Death rate	2	10.52%		
Number of patients with tumor recurrence, progression or residual IME	8	42.1%		

Abbreviations: CHT = chemotherapy; GTR = gross-total resection; IME = intramedullary ependymoma; MRI = magnetic resonance image; STR = subtotal-resection; XRT = radiation therapy.

Of the **intraspinal ependymomas (ISE)**, approximately 50% are **intramedullary ependymoma (IME)**, above the conus medullaris, and the remaining 50% are the **myxopapillary ependymoma (MPE)**, occurring in association with terminal filum, cauda equina, and/or conus medullaris. For anatomical and surgical reasons, these filum lesions are generally considered to be extramedullary tumors [14-16, 26, 35].

Abnormal signaling through the platelet-derived growth factor receptor (PDGFR) has been proposed as a possible mechanism of spinal cord glioma initiation and progression. The PDGFRα was seen to be expressed in a significant subset of these tumors across all major glioma types, including ependymoma, oligodendroglioma, astrocytoma and glioblastoma [12].

Table 2. Summary of the patients with myxopapillary ependymomas from the University of Wisconsin Hospital series

MYXOPAPILLARY EPENDYMOMA		
MPE	Number (N)	Percentage (%)
Number of patients	19	100%
Grade I (MPE) neoplasm	19	100%
Location in the spine		
Number of regions affected in the spine	33	100%
Cervico-medullary	0	0
Cervical	2	6.06%
Thoracic	5	15.15%
Lumbar (lumbosacral/cauda equina/terminal filum region)	17	51.51%
Sacral	3	9.09%
Multiple locations and/or metastasis	3	
Gender		
Male	15	78.94%
Female	4	21.05%
Coexisting neoplastic condition		
CNS neoplasms	0	0
Other neoplasms	4	21.05%
Neurofibromatosis type I (NF I)	0	0
Neurofibromatosis type II (NF II)	0	0
Other relevant spinal disease	4	21.05%
Age		
Mean age	50.92 years	
Range	26.64 to 77.91 years	
Clinical scenario		
Axial pain	18	94.73%
Radicular and/or referred pain	13	68.42%
Motor deficit	6	31.57%
Sensory deficit	10	52.63%
Coordination and/or balance	1	5.26%
Gait difficult	1	5.26%
Urinary disturbance	6	31.57%
Rectal disturbance	1	5.26%
Sexual dysfunction	4	21.01%

Table 2. (Continued)

MYXOPAPILLARY EPENDYMOMA				
MPE	**Number (N)**	**Percentage (%)**		
Spinal deformity	1	5.26%		
Mean duration of symptoms (before the 1st surgery)	22.06 months			
Diagnostic testing				
Preoperative MRI of the involved area	19	100%		
Postoperative MRI of the involved area	19	100%		
Eletroneuromiography	5	26.31%		
Treatment of the MPE				
Spinal surgery approach				
Patients operated for MPE		19		
Surgical procedures to remove the tumor	25	100%		
Posterior or posterolateral approach	25	100%		
Laminectomy	22	88%		
Laminoplasty	3	12%		
Posterolateral fusion	1	4%		
Anterior or anterolateral approach	0	0		
Combined approach (front and back)	0	0		
Postoperative neurological result (last surgery)				
Unchanged	13	68.42%		
Improved	4	21.05%		
Deteriorated	2	10.52%		
McCormick functional grade (last surgery)	I	II	III	IV
Before surgery	12	7	0	0
Immediate after surgery	13	4	2	0
3 months after surgery	12	6	1	0
1 year after surgery	12	6	1	0
Latest follow-up (from the last surgery)	12	5	1	1
Mean follow-up (from the last surgery)	29.01 months			
Radiation therapy for MPE				
Patients submitted to XRT	5	26.25%		
Complication related to the XRT	0	0		
Chemotherapy for MPE				
Patients submitted to CHT	0	0		
Number of CHT	0	0		
Systemic chemotherapy	0	0		
Intrathecal chemotherapy	0	0		
Postoperative mortality (period)				
Short term (<1 month)				
Intraoperative	0	0		
<1 month	0	0		
Medium and long term	0	0		
Mean death period	0			
Death rate	0			
Number of patients with tumor recurrence, progression or residual MPE	6	31.6%		

Abbreviations: CHT = chemotherapy; GTR = gross-total resection; MPE = myxopapillary ependymoma; MRI = magnetic resonance image; STR = subtotal-resection; XRT = radiation therapy.

This chapter utilized the WHO classification of tumors of the central nervous system (CNS) to distinguish the various clinico-pathological entities of the population studied. The CNS neoplasms are classified as: grade I (myxopapillary ependymoma), grade I (subependymoma), grade II (ependymoma), and grade III (anaplastic ependymoma) [30].

The series of 38 consecutive patients operated for **intraspinal ependymoma** at the **University of Wisconsin Hospital (UWH)**, Madison (WI), USA, published by Figueiredo et al. [15] was presented at this manuscript. Among those 38 patients, 19 had MPE and 19 IME, treated at the UWH, between January 1998 and January 2012. Patient socio-demographic data, clinical relevant alterations, tumor histological characteristics, diagnostics studies, treatment modalities, surgical techniques and complications, functional classification scheme (McCormick clinical/functional classification) [35], tumor recurrence and patient survival were discussed (Tables 1-2).

This chapter is also based on a contemporary **review** of the **literature** and on an **evidence-based systematic review** about **intraspinal ependymoma** published by Figueiredo et al. [16], concerning **MPE** and **IME**. The evidence-based systematic review of the literature proposes guidelines for the management of patients with ISE. The search was performed using the PubMed (indexed for MEDLINE), and Cochrane Database of Systematic Reviews, limited to articles regarding intraspinal ependymomas. The exclusion of case series before 2002 was aiming to reflect more current practices using modern imaging techniques, use of microsurgery, ultrasonic aspirator, intraoperative ultrasonography, image based neuronavigation, and intraoperative neurophysiology for the treatment of ISE (Tables 3-4).

Table 3. Evidence-based systematic review - quantitative summary of the papers related to intramedullary ependymoma

Characteristics	Description (after systematic review)
Papers	• 4 papers (included)
Study description	• All retrospective studies
Patients (n)	• Total number = **143** patients
Patients per study	• Mean = **35.75 patients/study**
Age	• Mean age = **42.72** years • Specified = 75% (3/4) of the articles
Gender	• **Male = 64.54%** (71/110) of the patients • **Female = 35.45%** (39/110) of the patients • Specified = 75% (3/4) of the articles
Tumor location	• **C-medullary = 1.81%** (2/110) of the patients • **C = 67.27%** (74/110) of the patients • **CT = 4.54%** (5/110) of the patients • **T = 24.54%** (27/110) of the patients • **TL = 1.81%** (2/110) of the patients • **LS/conus = 6.36%** (7/110) of the patients • **Cauda equina/terminal filum = 0%** (0/110) of the patients • Specified = 75% (3/4) of the articles
Histology	• **Grade II = 100%** (143/143) of the patients

Table 3. (Continued)

Characteristics	Description (after systematic review)
Clinical scenario	• **Pain = 66.36%** (73/110) of the patients • **Motor deficit = 62.72%** (69/110) of thepatients • **Sensory deficit = 57.27%** (63/110) of the patients • **Urinary/rectal incontinence = 30%** (33/110) of the patients • **Neurofibromatosis (type 2) = 3.63%** (4/110) of the patients • Specified = 75% (3/4) of the articles
Duration of symptoms (previous to the treatment)	• **Mean = 19.85 months** • Specified = 75% (3/4) of the articles
Characteristics	**Description (after systematic review)**
Follow-up	• **Mean = 25.1 months** • Specified = 50% (2/4)
Pre and postoperative clinical evaluation	• Clinical (pre-treatment) **assessment** used **McCormick scale = 50% (2/4)** of the articles • **ASIA = 25%** (1/4) of the articles • **Frankel = 25%** (1/4) of the articles
Postoperative neurological status	• **Unchanged = 61.53%** (16/26) of the patients • **Improved = 26.92%** (7/26) of the patients • **Worsened = 11.53%** (3/26) of the patients • Specified = 75% (3/4) of the articles • Described = 18.18% (26/143) of the patients
Surgery (initial)	• **Posterior/posterolateral** approach = **100%** (143) of the patients • Specified = 100% (4/4) of the articles • **Laminectomy = 48.18%** (53/110) of the patients • **Laminoplasty = 36.36%** (40/110) of the patients • Specified = 75% (3/4) of the articles
Surgical removal (initial)[22]	• **GTR** (100%) = **83.21%** (119/143) of the patients • **STR** (80-99%) = **14.68%** (/143) of the patients • **Partial** (50-79%) = **0.69%** (1/143) of the patients • **Biopsy** (<50%) = **0.69%** (1/143) of the patients • According to the surgeon report and/or <1 month postoperative MRI • Specified = 100% (4/4) of the articles • Specified = 100% (143/143) of the patients
Special surgical **equipment**	• Use of **microscope** • Reported use of microscope (after 1990s) = **100%** (4/4) of the articles • Intraoperative **neuromonitoring** (INM) • Reported use of INM (after 1990s) = **89.51%** (128/143) of the patients • **SSEP = 89.51%** (128/143) of the patients • **MEP = 8.39%** (12/143) of the patients • Intraoperative **ultrasound** (IUS) • Reported use of IUS (after 1990s) = "some patients" • **Ultrasonic** Surgical **Aspirator** (CUSA or similar) Reported use of CUSA (after 1990s) = **0%**

Characteristics	Description (after systematic review)
	• Surgical **laser** (SL) Reported use of SL (after 1990s) = 0% • Specified the special equipment utilized = 100% (4/4) of the articles
Clinical post-treatment **complications**	• **Complication rate = 32.72%** (36/110) of the patients • Main complications described **Urinary tract infection = 8%** (4/50) of the patients • **CSF leak = 8% (4/50)** of the patients • **Hematoma = 6% (3/50)** of the patients • **DVT/PE = 6% (3/50)** of the patients • **Pneumonia = 4% (2/50)** of the patients • Specified = 75% (3/4) of the articles
Radiotherapy	• **XRT used = 20.9%** (23/110) of the patients • Specified = 75% (3/4) of the articles Main **indications** After incomplete resection and/or recurrence and/or disease progression = **100%** (4/4) • Specified = 100% (4/4) of the articles • Mean **XRT dose** = 54 Gy **High dose (≥50 Gy) = 100%** (1/1) • Low dose (<50 Gy) = 0% • Specified = 25% (1/4) of the articles XRT technique or volume technique were not specified
Chemotherapy	• **CHT used = 1.81%** (2/110) of the patients • Salvage treatment = 100% (2/2) of the patients • Specified = 75% (3/4) of the articles
Tumor **recurrence**	• Overall **recurrence rate** = **3.63%** (4/110) of the patients • Specified = 75% (3/4) of the articles • Recurrence rate according to **treatment** • **STR** alone = **5.26%** (1/19) of the patients • **GTR** alone = **3.37%** (3/89) of the patients • Specified = 75% (3/4) of the articles • Mean 5 or 10 years PFS were not described
Death and cause	• Total **death rate** = **2.09%** (3/143) • Main **causes** • **Tumor related** = **0%** • **Other** and unknown causes = **100%** (3/3) • Specified = 100% (126/126) of the patients

Abbreviations: ASIA = American Spine Injury Association; C = cervical; CM = cervico-medullary; CT = cervicothoracic; CT = computed tomography; CHT = chemotherapy; CSF = cerebrospinal fluid; CUSA = Cavitron Ultrasonic Surgical Aspirator; DVT = deep vein thrombosis; GTR = gross-total resection; IME = intramedullary ependymoma (cellular); INM = Intraoperative neuromonitoring; ISE = intraspinal ependymoma; IUS = Intraoperative ultrasound; KPS = Karnofski Performance Score; L = lumbar; LS = lumbosacral; MEP = motor evoked potential; MPE = myxopapillary ependymoma; MRI = magnetic resonance image; OS = overall survival; PE = pulmonary embolism; PFS = Progression-free survival; PO = Postoperative; SL = Surgical laser; SSEP = somatosensory evoked potential; STR = subtotal-resection; T = thoracic; TL = thoracolumbar; XTR = radiation therapy.

According to the **evidence-based systematic review** about **intraspinal ependymoma**, the histological subtypes encountered were: grade I (myxopapillary ependymoma) in 57.03%, grade I (subependymoma) in 0.58%, grade II (ependymoma) in 40.61%, and grade III (anaplastic ependymoma) in 1.31% [16] (Tables 3-4).

Intramedullary and myxopapillary ependymoma are two quite distinct pathological entities, regarding biological behaviour, clinico-epidemiological data, management and outcome, and for this reason, we will present it separately in this chapter.

Table 4. Evidence-based systematic review - quantitative summary of the papers related to myxopapillary ependymoma

Characteristics	Description (after systematic review)
Papers	• 5 papers (included)
Study description	• All retrospective studies
Patients (n)	• Total number = **199 patients**
Patients per study	• Mean = **39.8 patients/study**
Age	• Mean age = **39.25 years** • Specified = 80% (4/5) of the articles
Gender	• **Male = 50.75%** (101/199) patients • **Female = 49.24%** (98/199) patients • Specified = 100% (5/5) of the articles
Tumor location	• **CT = 2.51%** (5/199) of the patients • **T = 5.02%** (10/199) of the patients • **TL = 24.62%** (49/199) of the patients • **LS/conus/cauda equina/terminal filum = 68.84%** (137/199) of the patients • Specified = 100% (5/5) of the articles
Histology	• **Grade I (MPE) = 100%** (5/5) of the patients
Clinical scenario	• **Pain = 87.93%** (153/174) of the patients • **Sensory deficit = 54.02%** (94/174) of the patients • **Motor deficit = 43.1%** (75/174)of thepatients • **Urinary/rectal incontinence = 30.45%** (53/174) of the patients • **Gait disturbance = 20.68%** (36/174) of the patients • Specified = 80% (4/5) of the articles
Duration of symptoms (previous to the treatment)	• **Mean = 18.66 months** • Specified = 40% (2/5)
Follow-up	• **Mean = 96.3 months** • Specified = 80% (4/5)
Pre and postoperative clinical evaluation	• Clinical (pre-treatment) **assessment** used • **McCormick scale = 40%** (2/5) of the articles
Postoperative neurological status	• **Unchanged = 85.29%** (29/34) of the patients • **Improved = 5.88%** (2/34) of the patients • **Worsened = 8.82%** (3/34) of the patients • Specified = 20% (1/5) of the articles • Described = 19.54% (34/174) of the patients
Surgery (initial)	• **Posterior/posterolateral approach = 100%** (199) of the patients • Specified = 100% (5/5) of the articles

Characteristics	Description (after systematic review)
Surgical removal (initial)	• **GTR (100%) = 59.79%** (119/199) of the patients • **STR (80-99%) = 34.17%** (68/199) of the patients • **Partial (50-79%) = 3.01%** (6/199) of the patients • **Biopsy (<50%) = 1.5%** (3/199) of the patients • According to the surgeon report and/or <1 month postoperative MRI • Specified = 100% (5/5) of the articles
Special surgical **equipment**	• Use of **microscope** • Reported use of microscope (after 1990s) = **100%** (4/4) of the articles which mentioned it • Intraoperative **neuromonitoring** (INM) • Reported use of INM (after 1990s) = "some patients" • Intraoperative **ultrasound** (IUS) • Reported use of IUS (after 1990s) = "some patients" • **Ultrasonic** Surgical **Aspirator** (CUSA or similar) • Reported use of **CUSA** (after 1990s) = **50%** (2/4) of the articles • Surgical **laser** (SL) • Reported use of SL (after 1990s) = **0%** • Specified the special equipment utilized = 75% (3/4) of the articles
Clinical post-treatment **complications**	• **Complication rate = 21%** (25/119) of the patients • Main clinical complications described • **CSF leak = 11.76%** (4/34) • **DVT/PE = 2.94%** (1/34) • **Wound infection = 2.94%** (1/34) • Specified = 20% (1/5) of the articles
Radiotherapy	• **XRT used = 47.23%** (94/199) of the patients • Specified = 100% (5/5) of the articles • Main **indications** • After incomplete resection = **100%** (5/5) • After recurrence and/or disease progression = **80%** (4/5) • Specified = 100% (5/5) of the articles • Mean **XRT dose = 46.45** Gy • Specified = 60% (3/5) of the articles • XRT **technique** • External beam **(EBRT) = 66.66%** (46/69) of the patients • Conformational **(3DRT) = 23.18%** (16/69) of the patients • Stereotactic XRT **(STX) = 1.44%** (1/69) of the patients • Unknown = 8.69% (6/69) of the patients • Specified = 40% (2/5) of the articles • XRT **volume technique** • **Focal = 43.47%** (30/69) • **Non-focal = 40.57%** (28/69) • **Craniospinal = 8.69%** (6/69) • Unknown = 7.24% (5/69) • Specified = 40% (2/5) of the articles
Chemotherapy	• **CHT used = 4.16%** (5/120) of the patients • Salvage treatment = 100% (5/5) of the patients • Specified = 40% (2/5) of the articles

Table 4. (Continued)

Characteristics	Description (after systematic review)
Tumor **recurrence**	• Overall recurrence rate = **24.12%** (48/199) of the patients • Specified = 100% (5/5) of the articles • **Recurrence** rate according to **treatment** • **STR** alone = **100%** (2/2) of the patients • **Partial** resection + **XRT** = **100%** (6/6) • **STR** + **XRT** = **34.78%** (8/23) of the patients • **GTR** alone = **15.21%** (7/46) of the patients • **GTR** + **XRT** = **5.26%** (1/19) of the patients • Mean **5 years PFS** rate = **68.75%** • **Surgery** + **XRT** = **78.4%** • **Surgery** alone = **49.7%** • Specified = 40% (2/5) of the articles • Mean **10 years PFS** rate = **62%** • **Surgery** + **XRT** = **75%** • **Surgery** alone = **37%** • Specified = 40% (2/5) of the articles
Survival rate	• 5 years **OS** = **86.25%** • Specified = 40% (2/5) of the articles
Death and cause	• Total **death rate** = **10.34%** (15/145) • Specified = 60% (3/5) of the articles • Main **causes** • **Tumor related** = **73.33%** (11/15) • **Other** and unknown causes = **26.66%** (4/15) • Specified = 72.86% (145/199) of the patients

Abbreviations: ASIA = American Spine Injury Association; C = cervical; CM = cervico-medullary; CT = cervicothoracic; CT = computed tomography; CHT = chemotherapy; CSF = cerebrospinal fluid; CUSA = Cavitron Ultrasonic Surgical Aspirator; DVT = deep vein thrombosis; GTR = gross-total resection; IME = intramedullary ependymoma (cellular); INM = Intraoperative neuromonitoring; ISE = intraspinal ependymoma; IUS = Intraoperative ultrasound; KPS = Karnofski Performance Score; L = lumbar; LS = lumbosacral; MEP = motor evoked potential; MPE = myxopapillary ependymoma; MRI = magnetic resonance image; OS = overall survival; PE = pulmonary embolism; PFS = Progression-free survival; PO = Postoperative; SL = Surgical laser; SSEP = somatosensory evoked potential; STR = subtotal-resection; T = thoracic; TL = thoracolumbar; XTR = radiation therapy.

HISTORY AND CLINICAL DIAGNOSIS

The clinical presentation of patients with intramedullary tumors is somewhat variable. Early symptoms are often vague, and the progression of these tumors may be slow and subtle. In many cases, symptoms will be present for several years before the correct diagnosis is made. Pain, weakness, and numbness are the most frequent presenting symptoms. Pain usually localizes to the level of the tumor, and the distribution of the numbness and weakness corresponds to the location of the tumor within the spinal cord. Bowel and bladder dysfunction may also occur, but these tend to occur later. It is important that these symptoms be recognized as soon as possible to make the correct diagnosis and initiate the appropriate treatment, as patients with milder symptoms at the time of treatment tend to have a better overall outcome. In some cases, a more rapid progression of symptoms can be observed. For example, the growth of a metastatic or highly malignant neoplasm may cause a more rapid onset and development of symptoms than more benign pathologic types do. Furthermore, tumors such as ependymomas may haemorrhage, thereby causing sudden development of symptoms. The presence of fairly acute or subacute symptoms should increase suspicion for a non neoplastic process such as infection or myelitis [49].

Symptoms of morning back pain or back pain when supine often predict an intradural tumor. The cadence of development of a patient's symptoms can help with the diagnosis as well: a slow insidious course over a few months suggests a slowly growing intramedullary primary spinal cord tumor, whereas a more rapid course might suggest a metastatic focus of tumor in the CNS or an inflammatory disorder. The history and physical examination help narrow the diagnostic considerations in these challenging cases, but further objective data and investigation are almost always needed [49].

Complaints of back or neck pain are found in most of the patients with intramedullary ependymomas. Low back or sacral pain, leg weakness and sphincter dysfunction are the complaints and signs found very often in patients with myxopapillary ependymomas of the cauda equina region. Previous history is usually often long, because these tumors are slow growing and there are often mild objective neurological deficits. The average reported duration between the onset of such symptoms and diagnosis has been reported to be around 3.5 years [67].

As with intramedullary tumors, the clinical presentation of intradural extramedullary tumors can be quite variable. The location of the tumor can significantly affect the clinical presentation. Lateral location, as is common with the extramedullary tumors, can cause pressure on the exiting nerve roots, leading to local or radicular pain as well as segmental numbness or weakness. Once the spinal cord is compressed, a Brown-Séquard syndrome (i.e., ipsilateral weakness and loss of tactile discrimination, vibratory and position sensation, and contralateral pain and temperature sensory loss) can also occur. Ventrally located tumors, which are more common in the upper cervical spine, can cause a pattern of weakness affecting predominantly the distal upper extremities. Radicular symptoms can occur in the thoracic spine but long tract signs, including difficulty with ambulation and spasticity, are a common presentation. Although patients with tumors of the filum terminale and nerve roots of the cauda equina can certainly present with lower extremity symptoms or bowel and bladder dysfunction, the most common presenting complaint of patients with tumors in these locations is pain associated with recumbency. Back pain exacerbated with recumbency ought to prompt a search for a tumor in the cauda equine [49].

Preoperative and postoperative clinical evaluation can be performed to assign each patient with spinal cord tumor a clinical grade according to the **McCormick clinical/functional classification** scheme [35]:

- **Grade I**
  Neurologically normal; mild focal deficit not significantly affecting function of involved limb; mild spasticity or reflex abnormality; normal gait
- **Grade II**
  Presence of sensorimotor deficit affecting function of involved limb; mild to moderate gait difficulty; severe pain or dysesthetic syndrome impairing patient's quality of life; still functions and ambulates independently

- **Grade III**
  More severe neurological deficit; requires cane/brace for ambulation or significant bilateral upper extremity impairment; may or may not function independently
- **Grade IV**
  Severe deficit; requires wheelchair or cane/brace with bilateral upper extremity impairment; usually not independent

The **evidence-based systematic review** about **intraspinal ependymoma** was based on 27 papers, all retrospective case-series, included 1,211 patients operated upon for intraspinal ependymoma, including intramedullary and myxopapillary ependymoma subtype. The mean age of patients was 37.85 years, with slight predominance of male gender (52.49%). The most common anatomical area affected were the lumbosacral-filum terminal region (33.92%), cervical (27.9%), and thoracic segment of the spine (19.92%). Pain was the predominant symptom in most of the patients (74.17%), followed by motor (47.64%) and sensory deficit (41.88%). The mean duration of the symptoms before the surgery was 18.16 months, and the mean follow-up was 94.63 months [16] (Tables 1-2).

Intramedullary Ependymomas

A large population-based cancer registry (Surveillance, Epidemiology, and End Results study) has reported that ependymomas are more common in the spinal cord than in intracranial regions across all age groups (36.2% spine, 22.2% infratentorial, and 11.8% supratentorial), occurring more often in males (56.9%) [37].

In the series of Klekamp et al. [25], 79 operated ependymomas were included. They presented at an average age of 43 years (range 8–74 years) after a quite variable history ranging from 1 month to 12 years (mean 30 months), and an similar sex distribution. Pain and gait ataxia were the commonest initial symptoms. By the time of surgery, gait ataxia was the major concern for 43% of patients. Compared to the second major group of intramedullary tumors (i.e., astrocytomas), there were no significant differences detectable. Quite often, small tumor haemorrhages can be observed on MRI, particularly at the tumor poles. Usually, such haemorrhages remain clinically insignificant as long as they are minor or the blood can accumulate in a pre-existing cyst. In terms of the spinal distribution of these tumors, 36 were encountered in the cervical cord, 38 in the thoracic cord, and 5 in the conus area; 65% of ependymomas showed an associated syrinx.

In the series of Kucia et al. [28] of 67 cases operated of intramedullary ependymoma, their mean age was 45.6 years, with a male-to-female ratio of 2:1. The most common location was the cervical spine, followed by the thoracic and lumbar spine. The average duration of symptoms was 33 months, with the most common symptom being pain and/or dysesthesias, followed by weakness, numbness, and urinary or sexual symptoms.

In the **UWH series** [15], 19 patients were operated for IME (Tables 1-2). The socio-demographic data is summarized below:

- Mean age = 41 years
  - Range: 14-84.4 years-old

- Gender
  - Female = 57.9%
- Most common spinal levels affected:
  - Cervical/cervico-medullary = 34.5%
  - Thoracic region = 34.5%
- The histological subtype:
  - Grade II (ependymoma) = 78.9%
  - Grade III (anaplastic ependymoma) = 21.1%
- Main symptoms:
  - Pain
    - Axial = 89.5%
    - Radicular and/or referred pain = 52.6%
  - Sensory disturbance = 36.8%
  - Motor deficit = 21.1%
- Mean duration of the symptoms before the surgery = 12.9 months

The **evidence-based systematic review** about ISE [16] included a review of series including patients operated for **IME** (Tables 3-4), based on 4 papers, including 143 patients, which main results are presented below:

- Mean age = 42.72 years
- Gender
  - Male gender = 64.74%
- Most common spinal levels affected:
  - Cervical spinal cord = 67.27%
  - Thoracic = 24.54%
- Histological subtype:
  - Grade II (low-grade ependymoma) = 100%
- Main symptoms:
  - Pain = 66.36%
  - Motor = 62.72%
  - Sensory disturbance = 57.27%
- Mean duration of the symptoms before the surgery = 19.85 months
- Mean follow-up = 25.1 months

Myxopapillary Ependymoma

In the series of Klekamp et al. [26], 29 ependymomas in 26 patients were encountered, and 26 operations were performed. Three patients with extensive MPE over several spinal segments rejected surgery. Patients presented at an average age of 36 years (range 13–57 years) after a mean history of 25 months. At presentation, 70% still regarded pain as their main concern, with 11% each naming gait ataxia or motor weakness as the major symptom. Only 7% considered sphincter problems as the main symptom, even though 52% did have some problems with bladder function. These tumors may contain haemorrhages and may even present with subarachnoid bleeding. Extramedullary ependymomas arise from the ependyma of the filum terminale. Histologically, the overwhelming majority are myxopapillary. The main bulk of the tumor is located in the lumbar canal below the conus medullaris. Extension in the thoracic spine was observed in 31% of cases, and 24% presented with extension into the sacrum. Some may fill the entire lumbosacral canal. These tumors may spread due to subarachnoid seeding, therefore, MRI of the whole neuroaxis should be performed to rule out this possibility.

In the series of Kucia et al. [29] of 34 patients operated for myxopapillary ependymoma, 14 were men and 20 women; mean age 45.5 years. The average duration of symptoms before diagnosis was 22.2 months. The most common symptom was pain followed by weakness, bowel/bladder symptoms, and numbness.

In the **UWH series** of 19 patients operated for **MPE** [15] (Tables 1-2), the main results are presented below:

- Mean age = 50.9 years
  - Range: 26.6-77.9 years-old
- Gender
  - Male gender = 78.9%
- Most common spinal levels affected:
  - Lumbar, lumbosacral, cauda equina, filum terminale = 69.69%
  - Thoracic = 15.2%
- Histological subtype:
  - Grade I (myxopapillary ependymoma) = 100%
- Main symptoms:
  - Pain
    - Axial = 94.7%
    - Radicular and/or referred pain = 68.4%
  - Sensory disturbance = 52.6%
  - Motor deficit = 31.6%
- Mean duration of the symptoms before the surgery = 22.1 months

The **systematic review** about ISE [16] regarding patients operated upon for **MPE** was based on 5 papers, including 199 patients (Tables 3-4), which main results are presented below:

- Mean age = 39.25 years
- Gender
  - Male gender = 50.75%
- Most common anatomical area affected:
  - Lumbosacral/cauda equina/terminal filum region = 68.84%
- Main symptoms:
  - Pain = 87.93%
  - Sensory disturbance = 54.02%
  - Motor deficit = 43.1%
- Mean duration of the symptoms before the surgery = 18.66 months
- Mean follow-up = 96.3 months

NEURORADIOLOGICAL DIAGNOSIS

Magnetic resonance imaging (MRI) has revolutionized the diagnosis of intraspinal tumors, also assisting the physician for the proper treatment of the neoplasm. In patients with suspected systemic diseases such as NF-2, and to rule out multiple lesions, the entire neuraxis should be examined. Patients unable to undergo to MRI, may require computed tomography (CT) with contrast or myelography for the diagnosis those tumors, exceptionally. Standard X-rays can be used to evaluate the bone anatomy, spinal deformity and stability of the affected spinal segment [25, 49].

High-quality, high-resolution, T1-weighted contrast-enhanced and T2-weighted MRI, with and without fat suppression, is critical in the diagnostic evaluation. MRI of the entire neuraxis is often needed to search for multifocal lesions. A complete imaging search of the nervous system can identify asymptomatic lesions, which can also help focus the diagnosis [49].

Intramedullary Ependymoma

Ependymomas and astrocytomas are the most common intramedullary tumors, accounting for more than 90% of the cases [27].

Kim et al. [24] described MRI findings of 43 consecutive patients with pathologically proven intramedullary spinal ependymoma and astrocytoma to differentiate those two most common intramedullary tumors. In patients with ependymoma, older age and a larger solid component were more often observed than in astrocytoma. Central location, presence of enhancement, diffuse enhancement, syringohydromyelia, haemorrhage, and cap sign were more frequently observed in ependymoma.

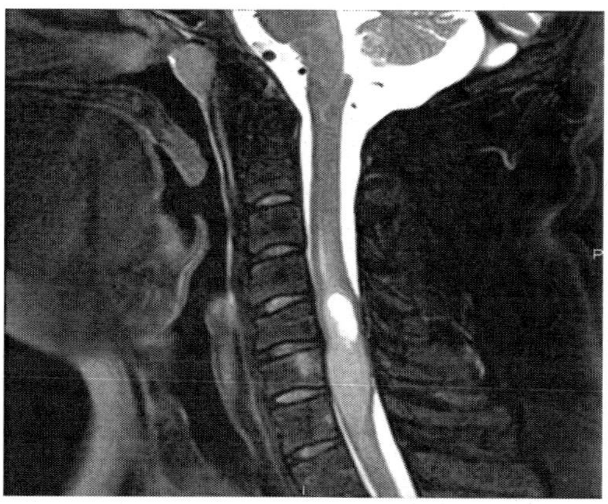

Figure 1A. Male, 39 y.o., MRI (T2 sagital with fat suppression) of the cervical segment of the spine, showing hyperintense intramedullary tumor from C4-7 spinal level, expanding the spinal cord. There is cystic lesion at the superior pole, mild spinal cord oedema just above and below the neoplasm. This feature suggests intramedullary ependymoma (IME), but intramedullary astrocytoma is also an important differential diagnosis. The diagnosis of IME was confirmed after surgery.

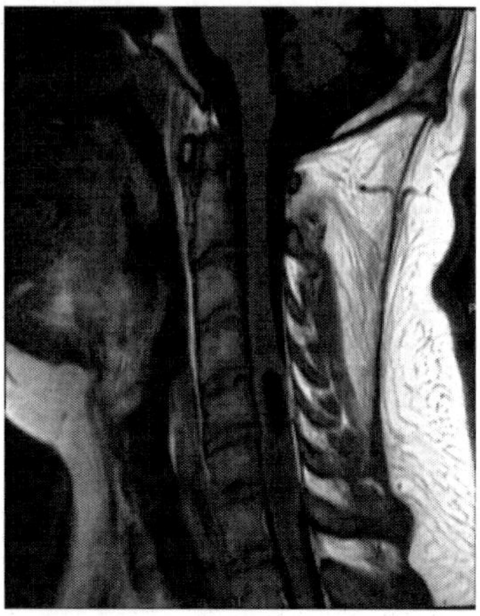

Figure 1B. MRI (T1 sagittal) of the cervical segment of the spine, showing hypointense intramedullary tumor, with cystic lesion with similar hypointensity of the CSF (cerebrospinal fluid), without clear limits between the lesion and the spinal cord.

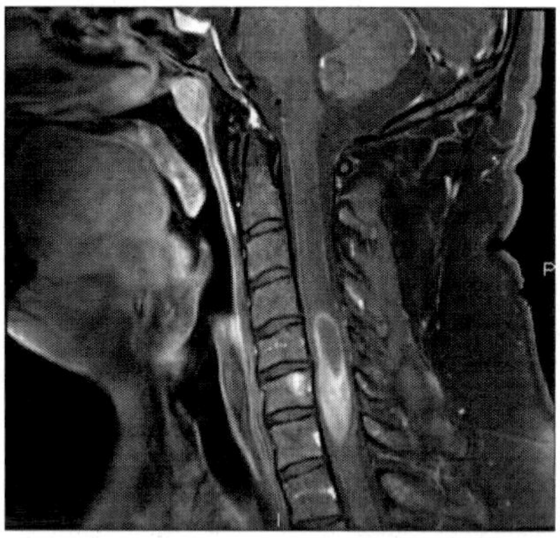

Figure 1C. MRI (T1 sagittal with contrast and fat suppression) of the cervical segment of the spine, showing an intramedullary tumor, with significant enhancement of the solid component. The enhancement of the margins of the cyst are features suggesting an intratumoral cyst, excluding syrinx and non-tumoral cyst.

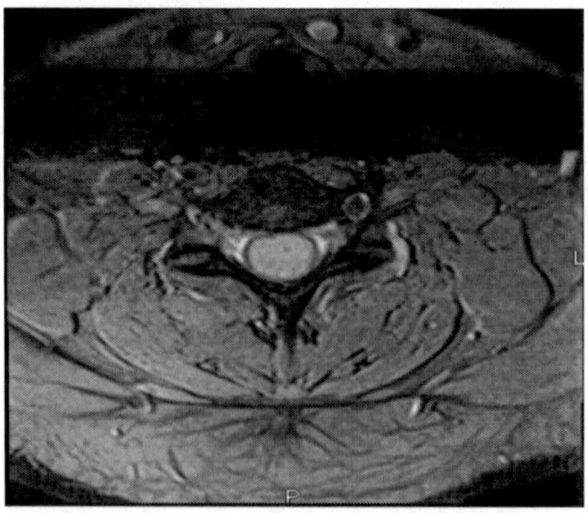

Figure 1D. MRI (T1 axial with contrast and fat suppression) of the cervical segment of the spine, showing an intramedullary tumor, with significant enhancement. The tumor involves almost the whole diameter of the spinal cord, which is visible as a thin layer of surrounding tissue at the periphery of the lesion, with intermediate signal.

The MRI has to demonstrate the precise spinal level of the tumor, including its upper and lower limits in T1 and T2-weighted images, and also the demarcation toward the normal cord tissue and precise location. Contrast injection is also mandatory, as the contrast enhancement is an indicator concerning the vascularity of the tumor and the homogeneity of the uptake may aid in the differential diagnosis. Inhomogenous uptake of contrast can be a feature of anaplastic or malignant neoplasm. The MRI can distinguish between a solid tumor and an associated cyst or syrinx [25, 61] (Figure 1).

The IME usually presents with a clear margin between the tumor and the spinal cord. Characteristically, the tumor is located centrally on axial images. It is often associated with haemorrhage as hemosiderin is deposited in the tumor. About 60% of ependymomas are associated with a cyst. On contrast Gd-DTPA (gadolinium-diethylenetriaminepentaacetic acid) enhanced MRI, almost all ependymomas enhance [21, 39] (Figure 1).

Myxopapillary Ependymoma

The three commonest intradural extramedullary tumors: meningiomas, schwannomas, and ependymomas, display almost identical signal characteristics: intermediate sign (isointense) on T1-weighted images and hyperintense on T2-weighted images [60].

Gadolinium-enhanced MRI is the gold standard for the evaluation of intradural tumors. Not only is MRI exquisitely sensitive with respect to finding even small tumors within the intradural space, but the signal characteristics on MR images can be very helpful in establishing the diagnosis for certain types of lesions, particularly lipomas, inclusion tumors such as dermoids or epidermoids, arachnoid cysts, and vascular anomalies. Nerve sheath tumors, meningiomas, and myxopapillary ependymomas tend to be enhanced after the administration of intravenous contrast. Meningioma may be the most uniformly enhanced of the group, although nonenhanced areas of calcium deposition may be present. Meningioma typically will have a more obvious area of dural attachment, the so-called dural tail, which distinguishes these tumors from schwannomas. Compared with meningiomas, schwannomas tend to be hyperintense on T2-weighted images. In the region of the conus medullaris and cauda equina, nerve sheath tumors and myxopapillary ependymomas may be difficult to distinguish radiologically. Both tend to be enhanced, but the pattern of enhancement may not be uniform because of the presence of intratumoral cysts, haemorrhage, or necrosis [49] (Figure 2).

Although myelographic and post-myelographic CT are not frequently used anymore in the evaluation of intradural pathology, those studies may be helpful in determining whether a lesion is intramedullary or extramedullary in exceptional circumstances, particularly when the patient has contraindication to be submitted to MRI [49].

Extramedullary ependymomas, like their intramedullary counterparts, enhance brightly with contrast. Enhancement may be homogeneous or patchy, as these neoplasms may be associated with small intratumoral cysts and haemorrhages [26].

Magnetic resonance imaging (MRI) scans reveal a well-circumscribed mass that is iso or hipointense on T1 sequences, and hyperintense on T2 sequences, with intense contrast enhancement [69] (Figure 2).

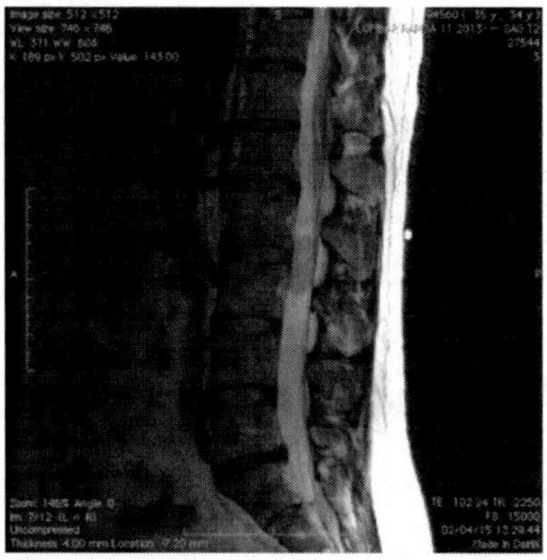

Figure 2A. MRI (T2 sagittal) of the lumbar segment of the spine, showing an oval shape intradural tumor, anterior to the nerve roots, at L2-3 spinal level, suggestive of myxopapillary ependymoma (MPE) of the filum terminale. The image also shows a degenerative disc disease of L5-S1. The diagnosis of MPE was confirmed after surgery.

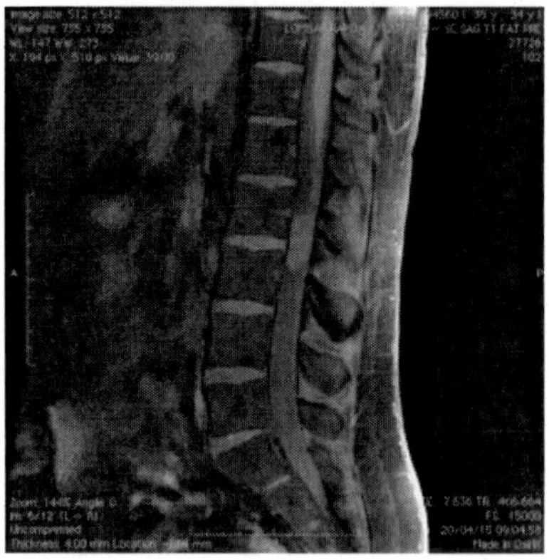

Figure 2B. MRI (T1 sagittal with fat saturation) of the lumbar segment of the spine, showing an intradural tumor, well defined margins of contour, and intermediate signal similar to the conus medullaris, suggestive of myxopapillary ependymoma.

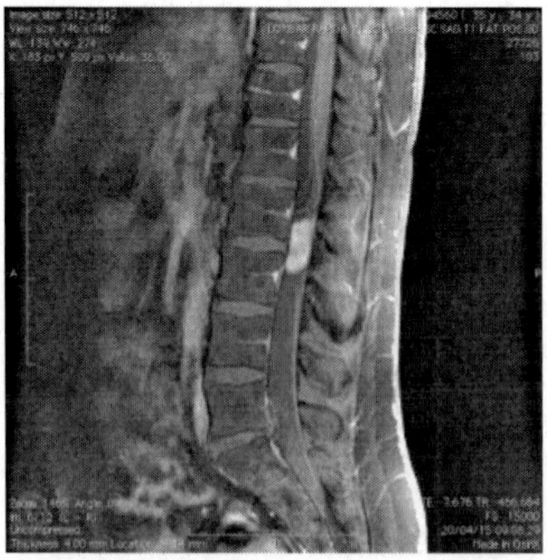

Figure 2C. MRI (T1 sagittal with contrast and fat saturation) of the lumbar segment of the spine, showing an intradural tumor, with homogenous and intense enhancement with contrast, well defined margins of contour, without extension into the dural surface, which suggests myxopapillary ependymoma, and excludes meningioma and extradural lesions based on the radiological aspects of the tumor.

The MRI for MPE typically shows a lesion in association with the lumbosacral nerve roots either as an intramedullary lesion of the conus or extramedullary of the terminal filum [21, 39, 57].

MANAGEMENT OF INTRASPINAL EPENDYMOMAS

Therapy for **intraspinal ependymoma** is mainly surgical aiming a gross-total removal, when possible without induced major morbidity, although even in these cases, the recurrence rate is 10 to 19% [8]. With complete removal of an intramedullary ependymoma, tumor recurrences are rare and the patient can expect a good prognosis. Tumor removal should be recommended as soon as the diagnosis is made, as the preoperative neurological status correlates directly with the success of the treatment [16].

We defined the **amount of tumor removal**, in accordance with previously published series [33, 41, 53]:

- **Gross-total resection** (GTR) = **100%** of tumor removal
  - Visible total tumor removal reported by the surgeon and/or at the control MRI performed in the first month after the procedure
- **Subtotal resection** (STR) = **80 to 99%** of tumor removal
- **Partial removal** (PR) = **50 to 79%** of tumor removal
- **Biopsy <50%** of tumor removal

Historically, complete macroscopic excision of these tumors resulted in significant postoperative morbidity and mortality, therefore subtotal resection with adjuvant radiotherapy was advocated as optimal treatment. Radiotherapy was usually reserved for recurrent tumors that cannot be completely resected and for malignant forms, which are rare in the spine. Advances in surgical technique, has led to reduced morbidity and mortality, and the role of XRT after intraspinal ependymoma surgery remains unclear, especially in cases of GTR [14-16, 35, 43].

Removal of myxopapillary ependymomas in the lumbar and sacral region may be quite difficult as these tumors are well vascularized and may not display a capsule, so that they may completely encase nerve roots of the cauda equina [26].

The surgical approach described at the **systematic review** about **ISE** [16] was posterior-midline in all the cases, being 83.54% through laminectomy, and 16.45% through laminoplasty, usually in the cervical region of the spine. The surgical microscope was used in almost all the cases operated on after the 1990s, and intraoperative neuromonitoring in 81.25% (Tables 3-4).

SURGERY FOR INTRADURAL SPINAL TUMOR

Preoperative and Intraoperative Care

After the proper preoperative and pre-anaesthesia evaluation and preparation, including the required images and tests, the patient is taken to the operating room. The surgery for intradural tumor is performed under general anaesthesia, considering the proper adjustments of the anaesthesia to be combined with intraoperative neuromonitoring. A Foley catheter is inserted. Intraoperative blood pressure is monitored with an arterial line, and mean arterial pressures (MAPs) should be maintained above 85 mm Hg throughout the procedure after induction of anaesthesia [10] (Figures 3-5).

Mechanical compression devices in the lower extremities are suggested in most of the **elective spinal surgery** to decrease the incidence of thromboembolic complications, according to the **NASS Evidence-Based Guideline**, as grade of **recommendation B**. The consensus states that for most commonly performed elective spine surgeries done through a posterior approach are associated with a very low risk of venous thromboembolism. In this setting, chemoprophylaxis may not be warranted as it is accompanied by a definable risk of serious wound and bleeding complications. Low molecular weight heparin or low dose warfarin may be used postoperatively to lower the risk of thromboembolic complications following elective combined anterior-posterior spine surgery, or in patients identified as having a high risk for thromboembolic disease, such as multiple trauma, malignancy or hypercoagulable state. These therapies should be considered carefully and on an individual case-by-case basis, as use may place patients at increased risk of bleeding complications. The consensus states that the mechanical compression should be initiated at the beginning of surgery and continuation until the patient is fully ambulatory is a reasonable practice [4].

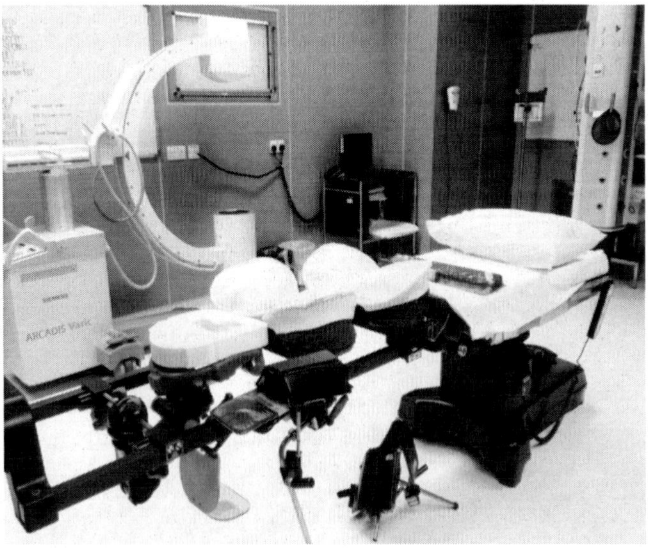

Figure 3. Operating room with spinal table ("Allen Spine System®") and standard fluoroscopic equpment.

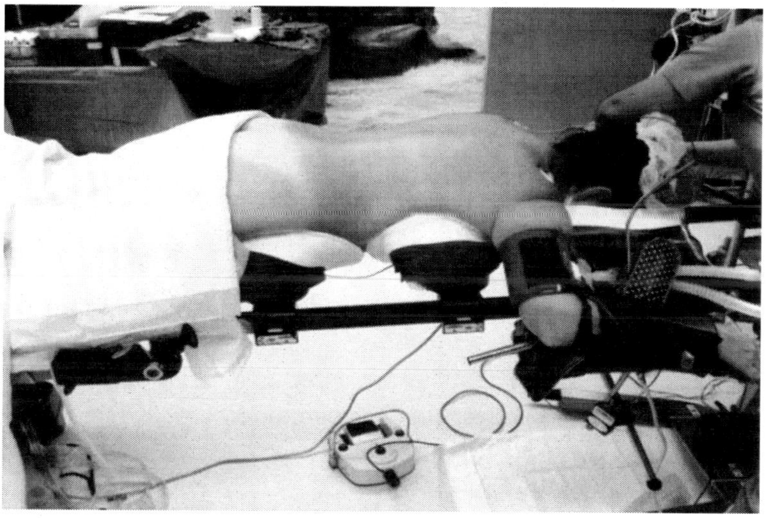

Figure 4. Patient under general anaesthesia, in prone position on a spinal table.

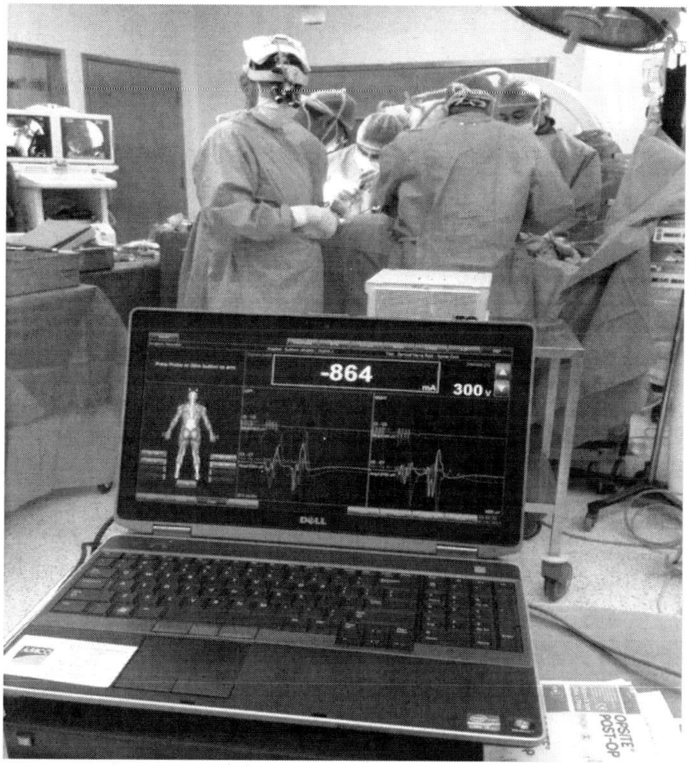

Figure 5. Intraoperative neuromonitoring equipment ("NIM-ECLIPSE™ Spinal System") during spinal surgery using surgical loupe ("EyeMag loupe" with LED light).

Preoperative antibiotic prophylaxis, with or without spinal implants, is recommended, according to the **NASS Guideline**. When determining the appropriate drug choice, the patient's risk factors, allergies, length and complexity of the procedure and issues of antibiotic resistance should be considered, as grade of **recommendation B**. The consensus recommends for simple uncomplicated spine surgery one single preoperative dose of antibiotic of choice with intraoperative redosing (at every 3-4 hours); and for instrumented spine surgery, prolonged procedures and/or comorbidities, one single preoperative dose of antibiotic of choice plus consideration of additional gram-negative coverage and/or the application of intrawound vancomycin or gentamicin [57].

For cervical and cervicothoracic neoplasm, the patients are positioned prone on chest rolls with a Mayfield or another similar head holder. For thoracic, thoracolumbar and lumbar tumors, patient can be place on prone position on a spinal table. The face is held in a prone view headrest with foam cushions, and the eyes are free from any contact or pressure points. The arms are positioned on arm holders with padding. The palms are placed in the pronated position, and the elbows are flexed at 90 degrees. The shoulders are abducted and externally rotated to 90 degrees but forward flexed to 20 degrees to keep tension off of the brachial plexus. Care should be taken to support the abdomen and thorax sufficiently to in order to limit epidural venous bleeding and to prevent pressure-related injuries during a procedure that will often take several hours. The spinal level of pathology can be confirmed by fluoroscopy before and during the surgery [10, 25] (Figure 4).

Surgical Technique

After being prepped and draped, a midline incision with a n°. 10 blade is then made from the upper to the lower limits of the spinal levels affected by the tumor, using magnification surgical loupes. This incision then taken down to the fascia level using a Bovie electrocautery device. The fascia is then divided to expose the posterior aspect of the spinous process and lamina of the area. A retractor is then utilized to pull tension on the muscular attachments to further the exposure of the posterior elements of the spine [10].

A laminectomy or laminotomy is performed over the spinal neoplasm exposing the dura mater. The craniocaudal extent of the vertebral arches removal should be larger than the durotomy, which should be larger than the tumor. For intramedullary tumors, a small medial laminotomy can be performed, about 10–15 mm wide. The vertebral arches can be opened with a small craniotome or a small diamond drill, and remove all laminae including the interspinous and yellow ligaments in one block. To avoid shrinkage of the interspinous ligaments, the laminae and ligaments can be stored under tension and moist with isotonic saline solution during the procedure. If a laminectomy is performed, the yellow ligament should be left intact during bone removal for protection, avoiding injury to the epidural veins. Once the vertebral arches are removed, the yellow ligaments are resected sharply. After removal of the yellow ligament or the laminotomy block, the epidural fat may be cut longitudinally in the midline and then mobilized laterally by shrinking it with bipolar coagulation. Quite often, however, epidural fat and veins are compressed and displaced laterally by the intramedullary tumor and veins will only start bleeding after the neoplasm is removed [10] (Figure 6).

Surgical Removal of Intramedullary Ependymoma

Prior to opening the dura, an intraoperative Doppler ultrasound ("Logiq E9™" [General Electric Company, Buckinghamshire, UK]) can be utilized to confirm that both the cranial and caudal apices of the tumor are visualized, especially for intramedullary tumors (Figure 7). From this point on, surgery is performed with the aid of the operative microscope, preferable, or with magnification loupes with the proper illumination devices. The durotomy is routinely made in the midline. The dura mater is retracted with 4-0 suture, which can be tacked to the fascia or paraspinal muscles. The arachnoid can be opened with microscissors [10].

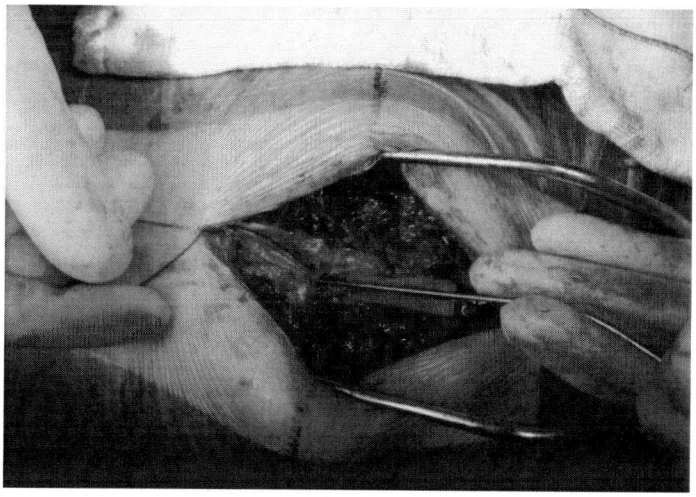

Figure 6. Posterior spinal approach for laminar opening and dural exposure during surgery for intraspinal tumor.

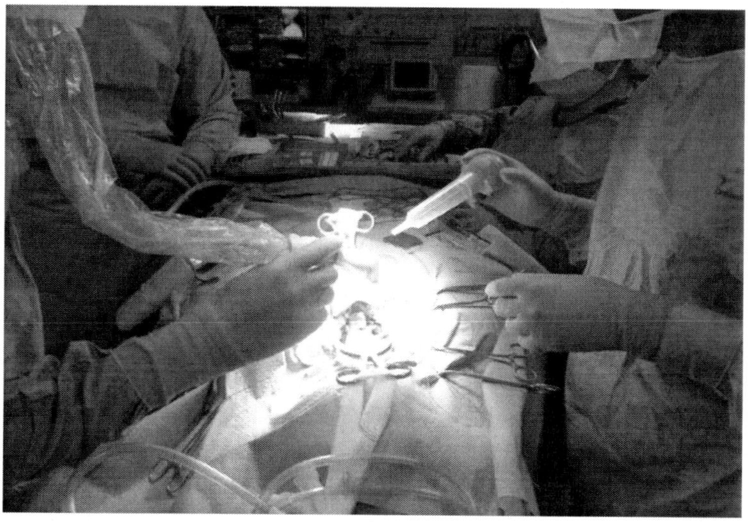

Figure 7. Intraoperative ultrasonography ("Logiq E9™", GE) for localization of intramedullary tumor.

We routinelly start the surgical procedure with the magnification surgical loupe ("EyeMag loupe Pro S®" with "EyeMag®" LED Light [Carl Zeiss, Jena, Germany]), 4.5 x 400 mm, and before opening the dura we remove the surgical loupe, and replace it by the operating microscope ("OPMI VARIO 700™" [Carl Zeiss, Jena, Germany]). After the tumor removal, intradural review, hemostasis and dural closure, we remove the microscope and we continue the operation with the surgical loupe again (Figures 5, 8).

Once the arachnoid mater is opened with microscissors, the spinal cord is inspected for a suitable area for opening. In many instances, the posterior aspect of the cord will not present any signs of the underlying tumor, unless the neoplasm has reached the pia mater or even grown exophytically. Sometimes superficial discoloration as a result of tumor haemorrhages may indicate the underlying pathology. However, especially in patients with an additional syrinx, the extension of the solid intramedullary tumor cannot be determined by inspection of the cord as the cord will appear swollen over a more extensive area. Therefore, the use of ultrasonography is suggested to check that the exposure is adequate and to determine the exact position of the solid tumor before the myelotomy (Figure 7). Basically, three options exist. In most instances, the myelotomy is done in the midline. If the tumor is located laterally, the dorsal root entry zone may be used. With tumors reaching the surface or those with exophytic growth, the spinal cord can be entered in that area. Care should be taken to avoid unnecessary coagulation of the posterior surface vessels, as this may cause significant sensory problems [25, 28, 31].

The reddish grey tumor surface of intramedullary ependymomas is generally quite distinct from the surrounding spinal cord, and typically a plane can be established completely around the tumor and the lesion removed in one piece. Occasionally, for large tumors, internal debulking may be required to facilitate dissection around the outer limits of the tumor [49].

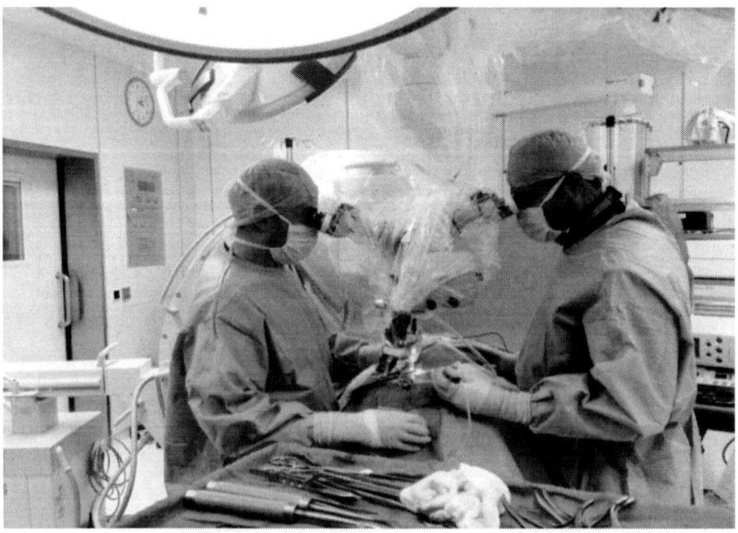

Figure 8. Microsurgical posterior approach for spine using the operating microscope ("OPMI VARIO 700™").

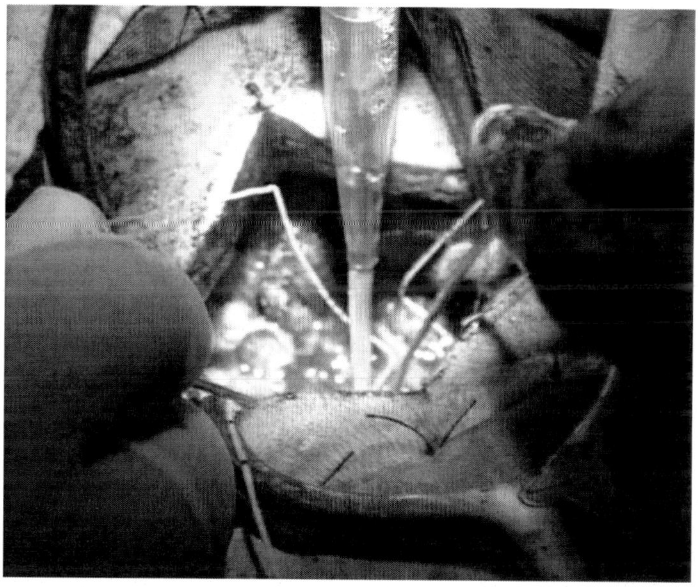

Figure 9. Ultrasonic surgical aspirator being used for the removal of the intramedullary tumor ("Sonopet Ultrasonic Aspirator").

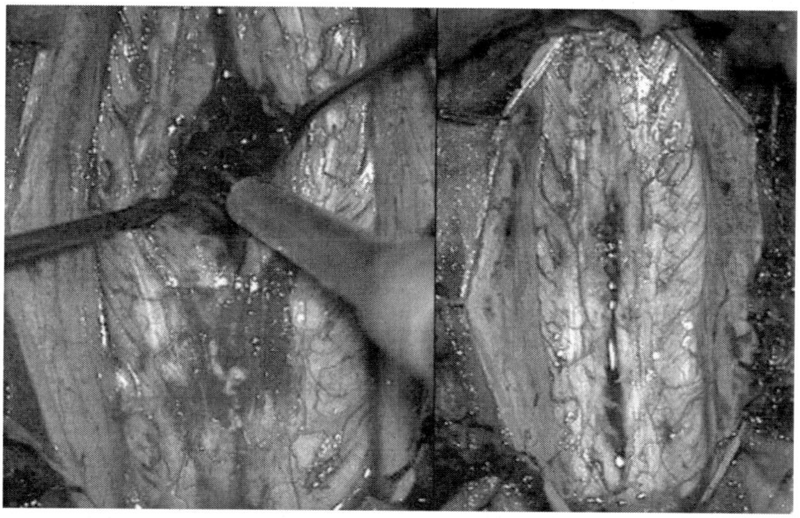

Figure 10. Intraoperative view of microsurgical technique for removal of intramedullary tumor through posterior median myelotomy.

The spinal cord should be opened over the entire tumor as the first step of dissection. A plane must be developed between normal spinal cord and the intramedullary tumor. It may be helpful to dissect above or below the apices of the tumor in order to find a clear cord-tumor interface, particularly if there is an apical syrinx or cyst. The plane is developed using microdissectors in the craniocaudal direction and then carefully around the circumference of the tumor. The tumor may be intemally debulked using bipolar cautery and suction, or ultrasonic aspiration ("Sonopet Ultrasonic Aspirator" [Stryker, Kalamazoo, MI, USA]) [10, 31, 66] (Figures 9-10). It can then be folded in upon itself to allow for further exposure around the periphery. Both frozen and permanent specimens of the tumor should be sent to the pathology for intraoperative and posterior definitive diagnosis, respectively. Once resection is completed, we achieve haemostasis with haemostatic matrix sealants and cotton micropatties. The dura is closed using a running 4-0 suture in a watertight fashion. A Valsalva maneuver is performed to confirm that no cerebrospinal fluid (CSF) leaks are present. Fibrin or a liquid adhesive can be applied along the suture line [10].

We close the deep, subcutaneous and subcuticular layers in the standard manner with sutures. Then, we use the liquid adhesive 2-Octylcyanoacrylate ("Dermabond®" [Ethicon, Inc., Somerville, NJ, USA]). The liquid adhesive should be gently brushed onto the incision, then, we keep holding the edges of the wound together for at least 30 seconds. After that, we apply another layer slightly larger than the previous one, completing at least 3 layers, with each successive layer applied after the previous layer has dried. The wound is not touched until dry, and we place a dry dressing over the wound ("OPSITE Post-Op®" [Smith and Nephew, HULL, UK]).

In the **University of Wisconsin Hospital series** [15], 19 patients with **IME** were submitted to 23 surgical procedures aiming to remove the tumor, and laminectomy was performed in 73% of the cases, as described below (Table 1):

- Posterior spinal approach = 100%
  - Laminectomy = 73.9%
  - Laminoplasty = 26.1%
  - Posterolateral fusion = 15.38%
- Intraoperative neuromonitoring = 73.1%
- Intraoperative ultrasonography = 30.8%
- Ultrasonic surgical aspirator = 30.1%

According to the **systematic review** [16], among those patients operated for **IME**, laminectomy was performed in 48% of the cases, as described below (Table 3):

- Posterior spinal approach = 100%
  - Laminectomy = 48.18%
  - Laminoplasty = 36.36%
- Intraoperative neuromonitoring = 89.51%

Myxopapillary Ependymoma

The surgical treatment of a myxopapillary ependymoma of the filum terminale should follow the same principles and basic surgical techniques described previously in this chapter for intradural tumors. The surgery for MPE depends significantly on the extent of the tumor and its involvement of the cauda equina. All patients suspected of having myxopapillary ependymomas should undergo imaging of the entire neuraxis to look for signs of CSF dissemination, which may alter the decision for a surgical approach. Ideally, a solitary lesion is identified in the region of the filum terminale without obvious involvement of the adjacent cauda equina. In these cases, the goal of surgery is gross total excision, which, if possible, should be performed *en bloc* to limit the dissemination of the tumor within the CSF [15, 49]. In these cases, the filum terminale can be identified both above and below the tumor. Electromyographic stimulation can be performed to confirm that there is no neurologic activity, and then the filum can be sectioned above and below the tumor, thereby allowing the tumor to be removed *en bloc*. Again, if possible, an intralesional approach should be avoided to limit CSF dissemination. Larger myxopapillary ependymomas with insinuation among the roots of the cauda equina present a much more challenging problem. These tumors can become quite large, and they tend to be unencapsulated and insinuated among the nerve roots. CSF seeding is a significant risk. Tumor resection in these cases is piecemeal, and gross total resection is rarely achieved. Although surgery may not be curative, it can confirm the histologic diagnosis and potentially improve symptoms in patients with large tumors [49].

Myxopapillary ependymomas are almost always found in the lumbar and sacral region. They may grow to enormous sizes, filling out the entire lumbar and sacral subarachnoid space. Due to the significant risk of subarachnoid seeding, extramedullary ependymomas should be resected *en bloc* whenever possible, together with the filum terminale [15, 26, 29, 49]. If debulking is required, this can be performed safely with well-encapsulated ependymomas, covering the surrounding surgical field with cottonoids and applying suction to avoid contamination of the subarachnoid space with tumor cells. Without a surrounding capsule, ependymomas tend to infiltrate nerve roots, making it much more difficult to achieve a complete resection without damaging important roots. Care has to be taken to avoid injury of the conus. The conus may be displaced and twisted, depending on the growth directions the ependymoma has taken [26, 29].

In the **UWH series** [15], 19 patients with **MPE** were submitted to 25 surgical procedures aiming to remove the tumor, and laminectomy was performed in 88% of the cases, as described below (Table 2):

- Posterior spinal approach = 100%
    - Laminectomy = 88%
    - Laminoplasty = 12%
    - Posterolateral fusion = 4%
- Intraoperative neuromonitoring = 80%
- intraoperative ultrasonography = 20%
- Ultrasonic surgical aspirator = 12%

The **systematic review** [16] among those patients operated for **MPE**, showed that the surgery was performed through posterior-midline in all the cases, but it was not specified if it was used laminectomy or laminoplasty, neither the use of intraoperative neuromonitoring (Table 4).

Intraoperative Neuromonitoring for Intraspinal Tumor

Intraoperative neuromonitoring is recommended and extremely helpful during all steps of intradural tumor removal [25, 31, 51, 62, 66] (Figure 5). The rationale for using intraoperative neurophysiological monitoring (IOM) is in keeping with the goal of maximizing tumor resection and minimizing neurological morbidity. For many years, before the advent of motor evoked potentials (MEPs), only somatosensory evoked potentials (SEPs) were monitored. However, SEPs are not aimed to reflect the functional integrity of motor pathways and, nowadays, the combined used of SEPs and MEPs in surgery for spinal cord tumor is almost mandatory because of the possibility to selectively injury either the somatosensory or the motor pathways. Besides standard cortical SEP monitoring after peripheral stimulation, both muscle (mMEPs) and epidural MEPs (D-wave) can be monitored after transcranial electrical stimulation (TES). Given the dorsal approach to the spinal cord, SEPs must be monitored continuously during the incision of the dorsal midline. When the surgeon starts to work on the cleavage plane between tumor and spinal cord, attention must be paid to MEPs. During tumor removal, monitor D-wave and mMEPs are important, sustaining the stimulation during the most critical steps of the procedure. D-waves, obtained through a single pulse TES technique, allow a semi-quantitative assessment of the functional integrity of the corticospinal tracts and represent the strongest predictor of motor outcome. Whenever evoked potentials deteriorate, temporarily stop surgery, warm saline irrigation and improved blood perfusion have proved useful for promoting recovery. Most of intraoperative neurophysiological derangements are reversible and therefore IOM is able to prevent more than merely predict neurological injury. Combining mMEPs and D-wave monitoring, when available, is the gold standard for this type of surgery because it supports a more aggressive surgery in the attempt to achieve a complete tumor removal. If quantitative (threshold or waveform dependent) mMEPs criteria only are used to stop surgery, this likely impacts unfavourably on the rate of tumor removal [51].

We use at our hospital the NIM-ECLIPSE™ Spinal System (Medtronic Sofamor Danek, Inc., TN, USA) equipment for intraoperative neuromonitoring.

Surgical Closure

Laminectomy has normally been used as a standard approach for intradural spinal tumors but this procedure may be associated with increased risk of spinal instability and deformity. Laminoplasty can be an option for the reconstruction of the spinal canal, where the laminae are fixed with titanium miniplates. Although it is still controversial, the main goal of the laminoplasty is to minimize the risk of postoperative complications, like progressive spinal deformity after the removal of the posterior elements of the spine. Laminoplasty was developed to overcome these limitations. Therefore, controversies still exist regarding the actual role of the laminoplasty in preventing spinal deformity in adults [25, 26].

Montano et al. [40] reviewed the data of 43 consecutive adult patients, who underwent either laminectomy or laminoplasty for spinal intradural tumor resection. Nine patients developed deformity or experienced a worsening of pre-operative deformity at latest follow-up. Among the considered potential prognostic factors, laminectomy and evidence of pre-operative spinal deformity were significantly associated with new-onset or worsening of spinal deformity. No CSF leak was recorded in the laminoplasty cohort. No new-onset spinal deformities, no CSF leaks and a lower rate of spinal deformity progression were observed after laminoplasty for intradural intra- or extra-medullary tumor resection.

McGirt et al. [36] studied the case of 238 patients undergoing resection of intradural tumor, including pediatric and adult population. Among those, 180 were submitted to laminectomy and 58 to laminoplasty. Laminoplasty for the resection of intradural spinal tumors was not associated with a decreased incidence of short-term progressive spinal deformity or improved neurological function. However, it may be associated with a reduction in incisional cerebrospinal fluid leak. Long-term follow-up is warranted to definitively assess the long-term effect of laminoplasty and the risk of deformity over time.

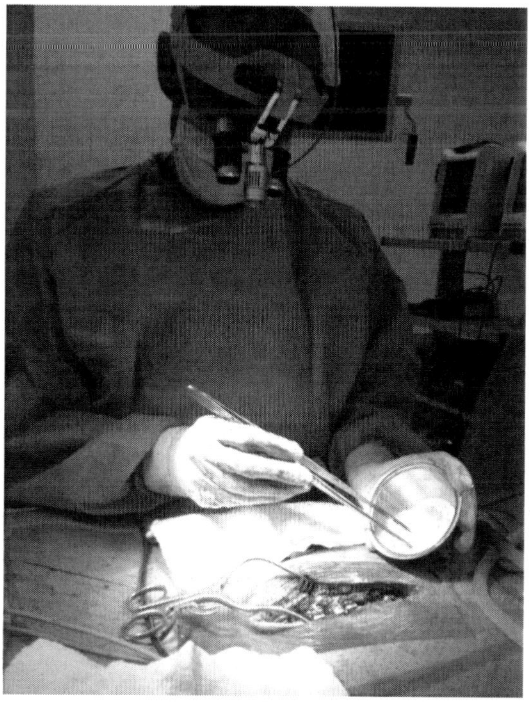

Figure 11. Application of intrawound vancomycin powder (1g) before closure (submuscular and subcutaneous spaces) during spinal surgery.

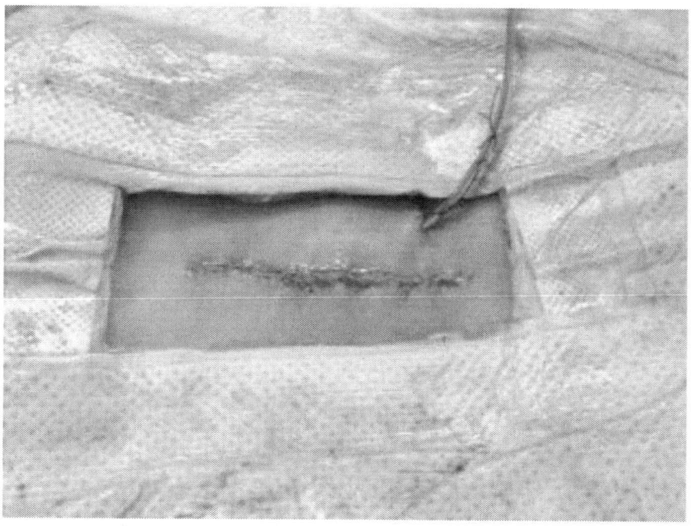

Figure 12. Final closure of the spinal wound with internal stitches, application of liquid adhesive ("Dermabond®") superficially and subfascial drain.

After the proper review, irrigation and haemostasis, local vancomycin powder can be applied to the wound before closure (500mg to 2g), increasing the local tissue antibiotic activity without significant systemic levels, protecting against surgical site infections by *S. aureus* after posterior spinal approaches [9, 23]. A subfascial surgical drain can be inserted, according to the surgeon preference, to be pulled out after around 24 hours, with an output inferior to 50 ml/8 hours. The wound is closed in the normal water tight fashion [10] (Figures 11-12).

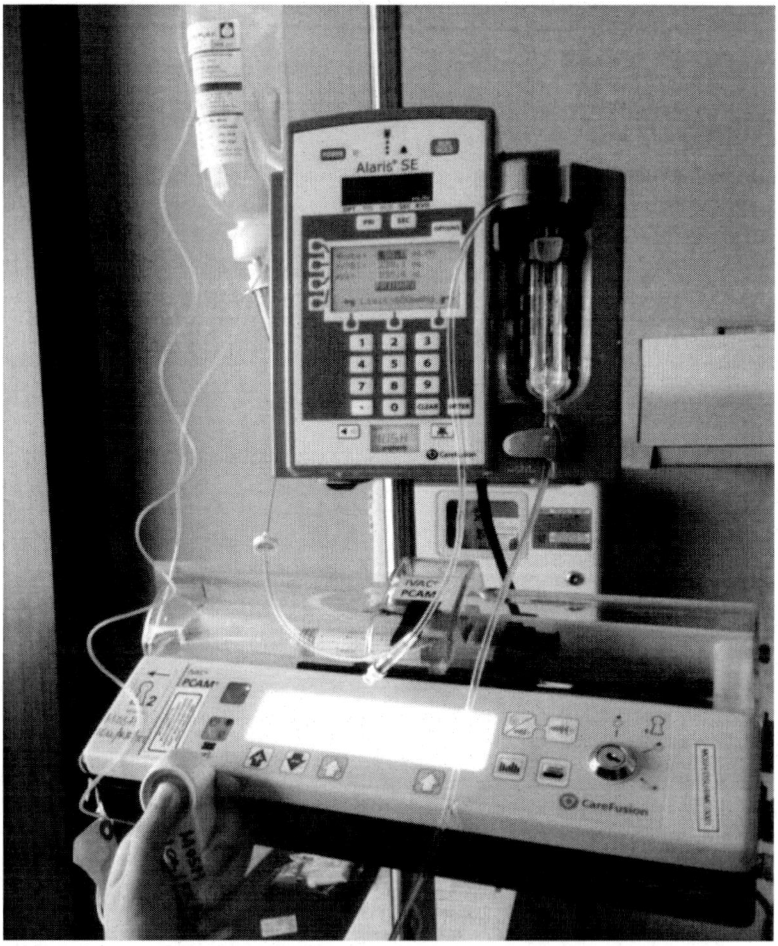

Figure 13. Patient controlled analgesia (PCA) using narcotic analgesics, like morphine, for the postoperative pain management after spinal surgery.

Postoperative Care

Patients with well-maintained dural closures postoperatively are encouraged to ambulate in order to prevent postoperative vascular or respiratory complications such as deep vein thrombosis and pneumonia. Orthostatic hypotension may occur after spinal cord injury secondary to tumor growth. This is thought to be secondary to the disruption of sympathetic activity control. This is seen more often after the resection of cervical or high thoracic intramedullary lesions and is thought to be due to reduction of plasma adrenaline and noradrenaline levels. These situations may be managed with fluids and gradual mobilization. Steroid therapy may be utilized after resection of spinal tumors although these should be limited to a short duration such to avoid the complications. The most common postoperative complaint after resection of an intramedullary tumor, besides the regional spinal pain, is posterior column dysfunction and motor deficits beyond baseline, which tend to improve with time. This is usually secondary to midline myelotomy required for tumor access as well as traction and manipulation of the posterior columns during surgery. This typically is manifested when the patients are ambulating such that they have difficulty navigating their feet due to a loss of proprioception [10, 45, 54].

While admitted in the ward, the patient should have the proper pain management, including the use of patient-controlled analgesia (PCA) with intravenous morphine (Figure 13) and anti-emetic drugs, soft diet, physiotherapy, anti-thromboembolic mechanical devices, and is encouraged to walk, according to the surgery and to the postoperative protocol. After discharge, patients should take oral pain medication, including acetaminophen and narcotic medications (both short and long acting), as well as nerve modulating medication (pregabalin or gabapentin). The patients are routinely seen during the first 2 weeks for the proper wound dressing, according to the case, and then, at 1 month, 3 months, 6 months, and 1 year, according to the follow-up. The result of the pathology should be discussed with the oncologist for the proper management. We developed some especific postoperative protocol for the main spinal procedures to be followed by the medical team and by the patient, and here it is presented the postoperative care after surgery for spinal tumor, where it is emphasized about the wound care, special to the risk of CSF leakage, among others, which is presented as follow:

Postoperative Protocol after Surgery for Spinal Tumor

General Issues

This is a surgery for removal (total or partial) and biopsy of spinal tumors, including neoplasm (tumors) affecting the vertebral column, intradural (lesions inside the sheath that covers the spinal cord/nerve) and intramedullary (lesions from the spinal cord tissue). These guidelines will commonly be associated with another one, according to the specific surgical approach for each case. Below is a list of general guidelines to follow:

- **Preparation before the surgery**:
  - The night or morning before the surgery date patient should take a full bath, washing the area to be operated with germ solution (2% or 4% of chlorhexidine or similar), applying it for 3 minutes (do not use brush), rinse and dry;
- **Extradural tumors** (lesions in the bone and outside the spinal cord/nerve sheath)
  - after surgery, the patient will begin to move carefully on the bed, and change decubitus carefully;
  - the next day, the patient can sit, get up and walk gingerly, with assistance;

- when the patient get home, can walk twice/day and may gradually increase the distance, according to individual ability and tolerance;
- **Intradural and/or intramedullary tumors** (lesions inside the sheath that covers the spinal cord/nerve)
  - In this case, the dura-mater (sheath that covers the spinal cord/nerve) is opened and closed after removal of the tumor, increasing the risk of cerebrospinal fluid leakage (fistula) at the postoperative period, what can cause spinal infection and meningitis;
  - after surgery, the patient will begin to move carefully on bed, and change decubitus carefully, but remain horizontally in bed for about 24-36 hours;
  - in the 2nd postoperative day, the patient can elevate the superior part of the bed (up to 45°), and stay in this position for 8 hours. If he fells headache or present with liquid drainage through the surgical incision, he should return to the recumbent position for more 24-36 hours;
  - if not, he can get up and walk gingerly, with assistance;
  - if he present with evidence of spinal fluid fistula, he may be taken back to surgery for additional closure and review;
- **General postoperative care after surgery for spinal tumor**
  - after return home, the patient can walk twice/day and may gradually increase the distance, according to individual ability and tolerance;
  - Sleeping and resting positions:
    - Lie on the back with a pillow under the lower neck and the other under the knees;
    - On sides, with a pillow supporting the head and another between the legs;
    - How to sit comfortably at 30-45° if using hospital bed (adjustable bed):
      - put the bed in a horizontal position;
      - patient lying on the top of the head at the upper limit of the bed;
      - rises first the hinge of the bed beneath the patient's legs (gaiter);
      - rises then the headboard;
  - Can take (full) bath after 5 days of surgery, standing or sitting, following the guidance regarding the surgical incision (to follow);
  - The use of pneumatic compression stockings (anti-thrombosis) in aid venous return is recommended for bedridden patients and postoperatively in order to reduce the risk of leg vein thrombosis and pulmonary embolism:
    - use pneumatic equipment while in the hospital bed;
    - use the compression stockings for about 2-4 weeks;
    - remove the compression stockings twice/day for 1 hour, and use it the rest of the time, including while sleeping;
  - Can climb stairs in moderation, since do not feel any discomfort;
  - Avoid bending, twisting the spine, or lifting heavy objects (over 5 kg) in the 1-2 months, and when need to bend, crouch with knees bent, grab the object, and lift with the back straight;
  - Do not drive a car during the first 1-3 months or while using medicines that may cause drowsiness or alter consciousness (derived opioids, muscle relaxants, and similar);

- Avoid physical/sports activities during the 2-4 months, except walk, until the medical release;
- Do not practice sexual activity for 2-4 weeks, according to the type of surgery performed. After this period, only if feels comfortable, with the back lying on the bed;
- Do not work in the 2-4 weeks, according to the type of surgery performed. After this period, only with the proper medical release, depending on the type of work;

Surgical Wound Care

The care of the wound is essential to prevent infection. Please follow the following guidelines:

  - Keep the wound clean and dry, avoid wetting it until the 5th. day after surgery;
  - If you want, you can take a bath protecting the operated region not watering it (involving plastic or avoiding washing that area);
- If used "Dermabond®" (sterile adhesive topic) or similar for surgical closure:
  - Do not wet, and do not rub or remove the adhesive from the wound;
  - After the 5th day, just remove the dressing ("Opsite®" or gauze), clean the entire incision with saline (or clean water + soap), dry it with gauze, apply the healing gauze dressing ("Fucidin®" or "intertulle sodium fusidate®" or similar) or oil ("Fucidin®" or similar) and cover it with "Opsite®" or gauze.
  - Repeat this procedure on a daily basis (or every other day) until the wound has healed well.
  - The "Dermabond®" should fall by itself after 2-3 weeks;
- If used "Steri-strip"® or "micropore®" for surgical closure:
  - After the 5th day, remove the entire dressing, and start taking full bath, clean the entire incision with saline (or clean water plus soap), dry it with gauze, cover it with "Opsite®", and thus the "steri-strip®" or "micropore®" that covers the remainder should also be carefully removed;
  - After exposure and washing of all surgical incision, dry it with gauze, apply the healing gauze dressing ("Fucidin®" or "intertulle sodium fusidate®" or similar) or oil ("Fucidin®" or similar) and cover it with "Opsite®" or gauze.
  - Repeat this procedure on a daily basis (or every other day) until the wound has healed well.
  - Avoid direct exposure to the sun;
  - If there are stitches in the surgical wound, contact the nurse and/or team physician for the proper withdrawal in about 2 weeks;
  - In case of suspected wound infection, contact your clinical/medical staff of the hospital for reassessment, follow signs that are suggestives:
    - body temperature above 38°C in 2 measurements at intervals longer than 4 hours (measure temperature twice/day for 5 days);
    - severe local pain, redness, swelling, opening of stitches, drain liquid or pus in the wound;

Management of Pain and Other Complaints

After surgery, during the healing process, there may be pain, numbness, tingling or even mild weakness in the operated region and/or in the limbs. While in the hospital, tell the nursing staff or doctor any of these complaints. Measures to be taken for pain relief:

- reduce activity and avoid sitting for long period for about 2 days;
- apply ice bag on the site of pain for 20 minutes at every 4 hours;
- use the prescribed medication, or any painkiller that is accustomed to use, as paracetamol or similar;

- In case of spinal fusion following the tumor removal (fixation of the spine with implants and bone graft), it is forbidden to smoke and the use anti-inflammatory in the first 3 months after surgery should be minimized (e.g., diclofenac, ibuprofen, naproxen, among others), since both impairs bone healing;
- Constipation is common in this type of postoperative, and should be reduced with the use of laxatives and diet;
- If these problems persist, or if in doubt, please contact the team, and/or return to the hospital/clinic for reassessment.
- Check routine first re-evaluation with the surgeon's office for about 1 week (for wound dressing and checking), and later around 30 days after surgery.
- Pathology result of the tumor biopsy has to be brought to the visit (please bring also the previous films and images).
- Most of the patients operated of spinal tumors will also need to be followed by an oncologist to the proper multidisciplinary management of the tumor.

These guidelines were developed by Dr. Nicandro Figueiredo, inspired at similar routines from the University of Wisconsin Hospital (USA)"

Surgical Biopsy

The intraoperative review of biopsy samples sent for frozen section is one of the most important tasks performed by the surgical pathologist. Proper tissue handling is particularly crucial at this stage of the patient's care. For almost all tumors, regardless of the sample size, 3 types of specimens are prepared: cytologic specimens, frozen tissue sections, and permanent formalin-fixed, paraffin-embedded tissue sections. In some instances, it is also prudent to place a small representative piece of tissue in glutaraldehyde for possible ultrastructural examination [49].

The intraoperative biopsy can be useful in certain circumstances, but should not be used as the sole criteria dictating the surgical objective. First, interpretation of tiny biopsy fragments often is inaccurate or non-diagnostic and may consist of only peritumoral gliosis, which may be erroneously interpreted as an infiltrating astrocytoma. Second, it is difficult if not impossible to accurately assess the nature of the tumor and spinal cord interface through a tiny myelotomy. Biopsy results, however, may be particularly helpful in some circumstances; for example, identification of a histologically malignant tumor independently signals an end to the procedure because surgery is of no benefit for malignant intramedullary neoplasm. In other cases in which the tumor and spinal cord interface may not be apparent, confident histological identification of an ependymoma reassures the surgeon that a plane must exist and that surgical removal should continue [44].

Special Surgical Considerations

In summary, the surgical approach should provide a corridor that completely exposes the tumor while minimizing disruption of surrounding normal neurovascular anatomy. In general, intramedullary tumors and extramedullary tumors located dorsal to the spinal cord are approached via a midline posterior corridor with the patient in a prone position. Extramedullary tumors located ventral or lateral to the spinal cord are approached via a posterolateral or lateral corridor. Often, these tumors compress the spinal cord eccentrically to one side. Therefore, a window of exposure can often be afforded through which internal decompression and debulking can be performed with bipolar cauterization and suction or ultrasonic aspiration (Figures 9-10). The portions of the tumor that were not initially accessible can then be delivered and rolled away from the neural elements for further resection. However, a clear plane of dissection between tumor and spinal cord must be developed prior to performing such maneuvers. Rarely, ventral tumors or ventrolateral tumors can be operated via an anterior approach. Intraoperative neurophysiologic monitoring including: somatosensory evoked potentials (SSEPs), motor evoked potentials (MBPs), and corticospinal MBPs (D-wave) are recommended [10].

The use of new advances in the neurological surgeries is strongly recommended to reduce the neurological complications, as the intraoperative ultrasonography, electrophysiological cord monitoring and microsurgical techniques [28, 31, 66]. Significant recovery may be expected postoperatively, with 80 to 90% of patients with incomplete neurological deficits showing improvement, even when the impairment is long-standing [17, 38, 42, 58].

Adjuvant Therapy

The treatment of choice in patients with an intramedullary tumor is surgery aiming at complete removal of the tumor. To perform a biopsy procedure with subsequent radiotherapy is no longer acceptable. Ifcomplete resection cannot be achieved, radiotherapyhas been recommended for ependymomas [26, 46, 68].

Radiation therapy is classically indicated for incomplete surgical removal, recurrence and for malignant histology. Ependymoma is a radiosensitive tumor, as a local dose relationship has been observed [46, 68].

Patients can be treated by different techniques and equipment for radiotherapy. The most used are with a ^{60}Co machine, 6-MV or 18-MV linear accelerators. The most common technique used is a single postero-anterior field, but some patients can receive 3-dimensional conformal and stereotactic XRT. Craniospinal irradiation can be delivered, usually for patients with leptomeningeal spread or recurrent disease. Local treatment is recommended for most of the cases to the region of the primary tumor, with 3-5 cm margin and a cone-down field that encompass the tumor with a 2 cm margin. The median interval from surgery to start the XRT is around 43 days (range, 14-140 days), median XRT dosage of 50.4 Gy (range,

44.2-60 Gy), dose per fraction of 1.8 Gy (range, 1.5-2 Gy), median number of fractions is 28 (range, 25-31), and median duration of 37 days (range, 23-65 days)[63].

The most commonly documented side effects of XRT are:

- Acute side effects
  - Skin reactions
    - Tanning and erythema
  - Gastrointestinal disturbance
    - Nausea, anorexia, and rectal symptoms
  - Fatigue
    - Weight loss
- Chronic side effects
  - Chronic pain
  - Neurological findings
    - Numbness, sensory deficit, extremity weakness, abnormal gait and sphincter disturbance
  - Hypothyroidism and premature menopause
  - Secondary malignancy [43, 63]

Intramedullary ependymomas are treated mainly with surgery, aiming total removal of the tumor, but adjuvant XRT is routinely given by most providers after incomplete removal to prolong PFS and OS. The systematic review of Oh et al. [43] showed a significantly prolonged PFS with adjuvant XRT after STR. Five-year PFS was improved by 20.2%, from 45.1% in the STR group to 65.3% in the STR plus XRT group. Most authors currently recommend doses of 45-54 Gy with long-term follow-up [18].

Myxopapillary and high grade ependymomas are more likely than other tumors to recur remotely and may be better suited to wider field irradiation to prevent recurrence. After irradiation, patients should be followed by MRI scans at intervals of once per year thereafter for 6 to 8 years because of the potential for delayed recurrence. Any recurrence should be treated with surgery, if possible, and postoperative radiotherapy [3, 32, 47, 59].

At the MD Anderson Cancer Center [63], adjuvant XRT is usually offered to patients with subtotal resection. Patients with gross total resection are often observed unless there are concerns about residual microscopic disease or concern for leptomeningeal spread. For patients receiving radiation treatment, the typical dose is 45 to 50.4 Gy at 1.8 Gy per fraction depending on location of the tumor. Although no standard dose has been established for adjuvant XRT after resection of spinal ependymomas, many investigators have used around 40 to 50 Gy.

The role of **chemotherapy** for intraspinal ependymomas still needs to be determined, and is being used mainly as a salvage treatment after recurrences and/or metastasis [26, 46, 63, 68].

In the **University of Wisconsin series** [15], 19 patients with **IME** were submitted to 23 surgical procedures aiming to remove the tumor, and some had also adjuvant radiotherapy, as follows (Table 1):

- Subtotal removal of the tumor plus XRT = 31.6% (6)
    - Complications related to the radiotherapy = 18.18% (2)
- Surgery plus XRT and CHT = 5.26% (1)
    - Due to simultaneous metastatic spread at the time of the diagnosis

The **systematic review** [16] of patients operated for **IME**, showed (Table 3):

- Surgery plus XRT = 20.9%
- Surgery plus XRT plus CHT = 1.81%
    - Mainly as salvage treatment after recurrence or tumor progression.

In the **UWH study** [15], 19 patients with **MPE** were submitted to 25 surgical procedures aiming to remove the tumor, and some had also adjuvant radiotherapy, as follows (Table 2):

- Postoperative XRT = 26.25% (5) patients
    - Subtotal removal of the tumor plus XRT = 10.5% (2)
    - Partial removal of the tumor plus XRT = 10.5% (2)
    - Biopsy plus XRT = 5.3% (1)
- Among those patients submitted to XRT there were no related complications, and no patient underwent CHT

This **systematic review** [16] of patients operated for **MPE**, demonstrated (Table 4):

- Surgery plus XRT = 47.23%
- Surgery plus XRT plus CHT = 4.16%
    - Radiotherapy showed a protective effect after surgery for MPE, even after GTR.

Results and Outcome

Intramedullary ependymomas provide in general a better prognosis than their intracranial counterparts. This is due to the fact that the spinal cord contains this tumor, the cord substance is displaced rather than infiltrated and, thus, the tumor is usually completely resectable with minimal risk of subarachnoid seeding, which is often observed with extramedullary ependymomas or ependymomas of the fourth ventricle [48].

Intramedullary Ependymoma

Ependymomas are completely resectable, in general, as they displace rather than infiltrate the spinal cord. Some ependymomas may exert such enormous pressure that they almost come out by themselves once the pia-mater has been opened. In such instances, the pia has to be opened quickly over the entire extension of the tumor and blunt instruments should be used for posterior and lateral dissection of the tumor. With an insufficient pial opening, on the other hand, posterior pathways may be injured by the extruding tumor. With ependymomas associated with a syrinx, the cyst may be lined by a gliotic wall. This gliosis can be left in place and has to be distinguished from tumor tissue. It is sufficient to remove the solid tumor part. The feeding vessels of the tumor have to be identified and cut, if possible, of particular importance are those arising from the anterior spinal artery in the midline. In any case, care should be taken to avoid too much tension on these feeding vessels as this may compromise spinal cord blood supply. Sufficient tumor debulking and coagulation and transection of these feeders are required to prevent such problems. Ependymomas may extend toward the pia-mater so that the dura may be exposed after a complete resection. In the absence of associated cysts it may not always be easy to identify the upper and lower margins of an ependymoma. In such instances the tumor may transgress into a fine thin structure towards the central canal. At that stage, this structure should be transected rather than followed further, which would require additional dissection deep in the center of the cord. Ependymomas may extend over several spinal levels and reach enormous sizes [25, 35].

Although spinal cord ependymomas generally have better prognosis than do other intramedullary glial tumors, factors affecting prognosis have not been clearly defined [20, 64].

Some studies indicate that older age and spinal cord tumor independently had better survival rates, compared with younger age and intracranial tumor (either supratentorial or infratentorial), respectively, although a consensus in prognostic factors has not been reached. Further studies identifying factors important for improving outcomes are critical to improve clinical management and prognosis. Ideally, an optimal treatment paradigm for an individual patient should be defined based on tumor features, such as histology, tumor location, radiographic findings, and presenting symptoms to provide optimal progression-free survival (PFS) and overall survival (OS) [37].

In the series of Klekamp et al. [25], 82% of intramedullary ependymomas were removed completely, while a subtotal removal in 15% and a biopsy procedure and decompression in 3%. The majority of ependymomas can be removed completely. Incomplete resections were associated with significantly higher permanent surgical morbidity (42% compared to 11% after complete resections, respectively), indicating lack of surgical experience as a major contributor to this difference. Complications occurred in 17%, with CSF leaks and wound infections as the commonest problems. Postoperatively, the majority of patients demonstrated an unchanged clinical picture so that early surgery is recommended.

In the **UWH series** [15], 19 patients with **IME** were submitted to 23 surgical procedures aiming to remove the tumor, and among those, 57% had gross total removal of the tumor. Considering the first surgery for tumor removal, the result was as follow (Table 1):

- GTR = 57.9% (11)
  - *En bloc* GTR = 21.1% (4)
    - All patients remained disease-free at the primary site at last follow-up (mean follow-up: 35.5 months)
      - Except one, which had postoperative XRT plus CHT due to simultaneous metastatic spread at the time of the diagnosis
  - Piecemeal GTR = 35.6% (6)
    - All patients also remained disease-free (mean follow-up: 39.7 months)
  - GTR (technique non-specified) = 5.25% (1)

        - Disease-free for at least 6 months
- STR = 31.6% (6)
        - Mean follow-up = 37.7 months
    - Living with stable disease = 15.8% (3)
        - NF II and multiple tumors had residual stable tumor = 5.25% (1)
        - Additional surgery (GTR) and XRT due to progression of the disease, living with stable disease = 5.25% (1)
        - XRT with stable disease = 5.25% (1)
    - Tumor progression = 15.8% (3)
        - NF II and multiple tumors = 5.3% (1)
        - XRT with slowly progressive tumor = 5.25% (1)
        - Deceased after tumor progression = 5.25% (1)
- Partial removal = 10.5% (2)
        - Mean follow-up = 23 months
    - XRT plus re-operation 3 times, and deceased after progression of the disease = 5.25% (1)
    - Living with stable tumor = 5.25% (1)
- Postoperative complications
    - Severe spinal pain = 23.1% (6)
    - Neurological worsening = 13% (3)
    - Spinal instability= 13% (3)
    - Urinary tract infection = 5.25% (1)
    - Wound infection = 5.25% (1)
    - Painful dysesthesia = 5.25% (1)
- Complications after XRT = 50% (2)
- Complications after CHT = 0
- Intraoperative biopsy discordant with the final diagnosis = 29.4%
- Postoperative neurological status (McCormick functional classification scheme)
    - Unchanged = 68.4%
    - Improved = 15.7%
    - Deteriorated = 15.7%
- Mean follow-up = 28.3 months (range: 1-85 months)
- Disease-free= 57.9% (11)
- Tumor recurrence, progression and/or stable = 42.1% (8)
- XRT = 31.6% (6)
    - All after recurrent, metastatic or residual tumor
- CHT = 5.25% (1)
- Deceased = 10.5% (2)
    - Death causes related to the tumor progression

The **systematic review** [16] about **IME** showed that 83% of the patients had gross total removal of the tumor, as described below (Table 3):

- GTR = 83.21%
- STR = 14.68%

- Partial removal = 0.69%
- Biopsy = 0.69%
- Postoperative neurological status (McCormick functional classification scheme)
    - Unchanged = 61.53%
    - Improved = 26.92%
    - Deteriorated = 11.53%
- Overall clinical complication rate = 32.72%
- XRT = 20.9%
- CHT = 1.81%
- Overall recurrence/progression rate = 3.63%
    - Highest incidence of recurrence in patients submitted to STR alone = 5.26%
    - Overall death rate = 2.09%
        - Not directly related to the tumor

Myxopapillary Ependymoma

Removal of myxopapillary ependymomas in the lumbar and sacral region may be quite difficult as these tumors are well vascularized and may not display a capsule, so that they may completely encase nerve roots of the cauda equina [6].

As extramedullary ependymomas are almost always found in the lumbar and sacral region, they may grow to enormous sizes, filling out the entire lumbar and sacral subarachnoid space. Due to the significant risk of subarachnoid seeding, extramedullary ependymomas should be resected in *en bloc* whenever possible, together with the filum terminale. If debulking is required, this can be performed safely with well-encapsulated ependymomas, covering the surrounding surgical field with cottonoids and applying suction to avoid contamination of the subarachnoid space with tumor cells. Without a surrounding capsule, ependymomas tend to infiltrate nerve roots, making it much more difficult to achieve a complete resection without damaging important roots. Care has to be taken to avoid injury of the conus. The conus may be displaced and twisted, depending on the growth directions the ependymoma has taken [45].

Myxopapillary ependymoma produce mucin and, by virtue of arborizing, form papillae. This mucoid matrix may render the tumor removal somewhat problematic [45, 46]. Pica et al. [46.] evaluated different potential prognostic factors regarding PFS in MPE patients treated with surgery alone, and surgery plus XRT. Their results showed that postoperative high-dose XRT impacted favorable on tumor control, increasing significantly the 5-year progression-free survival (82% vs. 50%).

Most articles on the clinical features and treatment of MPE have described the propriety of postoperative radiation and the tumor recurrence [41, 53]. Akyurek et al. noted that regardless of the extent of resection, adjuvant XRT significantly reduced the rate of tumor progression in cases of MPE [1]. Therefore, not all the MPE have so gratifying response to XRT, and irradiation may also causes myelopathy, which may lead to neurologic deficit. Data are very limited regarding chemotherapy for adults with intraspinal ependymomas, being reserved for patients in whom surgery and/or XRT is not an option or has failed. Reoperation for a previously irradiated lesion is usually more risky and difficult [41].

In series of Klekamp et al. [26], the overall tumor recurrence rates of MPE were 12% and 30% within the first year and after 10 years, respectively.

The MD Anderson report [63] demonstrated favourable long-term survival for patients with spinal MPE after surgery and adjuvant XRT. All recurrences were in the neural axis, mostly locally, supporting the use of local XRT. Patients who were older than 35 years of age at diagnosis had better PFS and LC than their younger counterparts. Adjuvant XRT provided PFS and LC benefit in all patients, after accounting for resection type in the multivariate analysis. The large absolute local control benefit of adjuvant XRT after gross total resection would argue for the use radiation at least in selected patients with gross total resection. Identification of such patients will require further study with a larger patient population with longer follow-up.

Among those cases with **MPE** operated at **UWH** [15], 19 patients with MPE were submitted to 25 surgical procedures aiming to remove the tumor, and among those, 73% had gross total removal of the tumor. Considering the first surgery for tumor removal, the result was as follow (Table 2):

- GTR = 73.7% (14)
  - *En bloc* GTR = 36.8% (7)
    - Disease-free at last follow-up (mean follow-up: 23.6 months) = 100%
  - Piecemeal GTR = 36.8% (7)
    - Tumor recurrence (mean follow-up = 25.7 months) = 10.5% (2)
    - Recurrence of the operated lesion and progression of multiple other non-operated tumors = 5.25% (1)
    - Tumor recurrence, submitted to a second GTR (piecemeal), and remained disease-free = 5.25% (1)
- STR = 10.5% (2)
  - XRT and living with stable disease (mean follow-up: 24.5 months)
- Partial removal = 10.5% (2)
  - Re-operated once plus XRT and is living with disease = 5.25% (1)
  - Re-operated twice plus XRT and is living with disease = 5.25% (1)
    - Mean follow-up = 84.5 months
- Biopsy = 5.25% (1)
  - Patient was referred to UWH after the biopsy for definitive management
  - Re-operated 3 times, submitted to XRT, and he is still surviving with stable disease (follow-up: 12 months)
- Postoperative complications
  - Severe spinal pain = 20% (5)
  - Neurological worsening = 8% (2)
  - Sexual dysfunction = 8% (2)
  - Urinary tract infection = 8% (2)
  - Spinal instability = 4% (1)
  - Wound infection = 4% (1)
  - Meralgia paresthetica = 4% (1)
  - Hydrocephalus= 4% (1)
  - cardiopulmonary disturbance= 4% (1)

   - Cerebrospinal fluid (CSF) leakage= 4% (1)
- Complications after XRT = 0
- Complications after CHT = 0
- Intraoperative biopsy discordant with the final diagnosis = 11.1%
- Postoperative neurological status (McCormick functional classification scheme)
  - Unchanged = 68.4%
  - Improved = 21.1%
  - Deteriorated = 10.5%
- Mean follow-up = 35.6 months (range: 1-92 months)
- Disease-free = 68.4% (13)
- Tumor recurrence, progression and/or stable = 31.6% (6)
- XRT = 21.1% (4)
  - All after recurrent or residual tumor
- CHT = 0
- Deceased = 0

The **systematic review** [16] about **MPE** showed that 59% of the patients had gross total removal of the tumor, as described below (Table 4):

- GTR = 59.79%
- STR = 34.17%
- Partial removal = 3.01%
- Biopsy = 1.5%
- Postoperative neurological status (McCormick functional classification scheme)
  - Unchanged = 85.29%
  - Improved = 5.88%
  - Deteriorated = 8.88%
- Overall clinical complication rate = 21%
- XRT = 47.23%
- CHT = 4.16%
- Overall recurrence/progression rate = 24.12%
  - GTR alone = 15.21%
  - GTR plus radiotherapy = 5.26%
- Overall death rate = 7.67%
  - Related to the tumor = 73.33%
- Mean 5 years PFS (progression-free survival) = 68.75%
- Overall 5 years PFS = 68.75%
  - Surgery plus XRT = 78.4%
  - Surgery only = 49.7%
- Mean 10 years PFS = 62%
  - Surgery plus XRT = 75%
  - Surgery only = 37%
- Total death rate = 10.34%
- 5 years OS (overall survival) = 86.25%

Discussion

Intramedullary tumors are typically derived from glial or ependymal cells that are found throughout the interstitium of the cord, being ependymoma the most common glial tumor of the adult spinal cord [44].

The treatment of spinal tumors has evolved and benefited from the general progress of the medical field and neurological surgery, especially with the new sophisticated imaging and with the use of microsurgery, bipolar cautery, ultrasonic aspirator, intraoperative ultrasonography, intraoperative MRI, image based neuronavigation, contact surgical laser and intraoperative neurophysiology, but these neoplasm still represent a challenge to the neurosurgeons and for the patients [56].

In a previous study, Schellinger et al. [52], using the Central Brain Tumor Registry of the United States (CBTRUS) database, which covers approximately 30% of the US population, identified 3,226 cases, with most common histological types being meningiomas (29%), nerve sheath tumors (24%), and ependymomas (23%). According to the biennial CBTRUS report, primary spinal cord tumors represent 4% of all primary CNS tumors [5]. Adjuvant XRT was usually advocated after incomplete resection, dissemination, recurrence or for the rare anaplastic ependymoma [7, 8].

Because of the relative rarity of these tumors, large prospective single center series are quite uncommon. It is important that institutions publish whatever data is available in order to better understand the biology, epidemiology, diagnosis, treatment and prognosis of these lesions, and to build evidence based consensus on the optimal management options for these tumors [11, 14-16, 28, 35, 43, 63]

Experience with patients having these **tumors** may be limited, even in larger medical centers. Yet, practicing neurosurgeons will encounter patients with intraspinal **tumors** and therefore need to be aware of their clinical presentation, diagnostic evaluation, types of **tumors** likely to occur, management options, and frequency of treatment complications [13].

Intramedullary Ependymoma

The systematic review of Oh et al. [43] aimed to evaluate whether adjuvant XRT has any benefit after STR of IME. A total of 348 patients underwent surgical resection of spinal cord ependymomas, where GTR was obtained in 77% of patients. Among those who had GTR, only 3.7% received adjuvant XRT, while among those who had STR, 58.8% have been submitted to XRT. The authors concluded that surgery remains the mainstay treatment for IME, where GTR provides optimal outcomes with longest PFS and OS. Adjuvant XRT prolongs PFS after STR significantly, and OS is improved by GTR and benign tumor grade only.

Kucia et al. [28] published their retrospective study of 67 cases operated of intramedullary ependymoma. Gross total resection was achieved in 55 patients and a subtotal resection was performed in 12 patients; 9 patients were treated with adjuvant radiation therapy. Mean follow-up was 32 months. A significant number of patients who initially worsened improved at their 3-month follow-up examination. Outcomes were significantly worse in patients undergoing subtotal resection with or without radiation therapy. There were

3 recurrences. The overall complication rate was 34%. The primary complications were wound infections or cerebrospinal fluid leaks. They concluded that IME are difficult lesions to treat. Aggressive surgical resection is associated with a high overall complication rate. However, when gross total resection can be achieved, overall outcomes are excellent and the recurrence rate is low.

In the **University of Wisconsin series** of patients operated of **IME** [15], it was demonstrated that GTR alone offered the best results, with no tumor recurrence. Subtotal resection also provided good results, but tumor progression and its complications were more common. Partial removal plus XRT offered a reasonable outcome, but with more tumor recurrence and complications.

The **evidence-based systematic review** [16] about **IME** showed that the best results were obtained in patients submitted to GTR, and the highest incidence of recurrence occurred in patients submitted to STR alone.

Myxopapillary Ependymoma

In the series of Kucia et al. [29] of 34 patients operated for myxopapillary ependymoma, the rate of gross total resection was 80%. All patients with a subtotal resection (20%) underwent postoperative radiation therapy. Presentation and outcomes of patients who underwent subtotal resection followed by radiation therapy were compared with those who underwent gross total resection alone. There was no significant difference in neurological grade between the groups at presentation or final follow-up. The overall recurrence rate was 10%. The goal of surgical treatment of myxopapillary ependymomas is resection to the greatest extent possible with preservation of function. In cases of subtotal resection, postoperative radiation therapy may improve outcome. If neurological function is maintained at treatment, these indolent lesions allow years of good function.

Tsai et al. [63] studied the role of radiotherapy after surgery for 51 patients with myxopapillary ependymoma. Twenty patients (39%) had surgery alone, 30 (59%) had surgery plus XRT, and one (2%) had XRT only. At a median follow-up of 11 years, 10-year OS, PFS, and local control (LC) for the entire group were 93%, 63%, and 67%, respectively. Nineteen patients (37%) had disease recurrence, and the recurrence was mostly local (79%). Twenty-eight of 50 patients (56%) who had surgery were GTR; 10-year LC was 56% after surgery versus 92% after surgery and XRT; the median time of LC was 10.5 years for patients receiving GTR plus XRT, and 4.75 years for GTR only. Among 16 patients with STR and follow-up data, 10-year LC was 0% after surgery versus 65% for surgery plus XRT. The authors concluded that postoperative radiotherapy after resection of MPE was associated with improved PFS and LC.

In the **University of Wisconsin series** of patients operated of **MPE** [15] it was shown that GTR was achieved in most of the patients, and *en bloc* GTR alone offered the best results, with no recurrence. Piecemeal GTR alone and STR plus XRT can result in long-term survive, but the tumor recurrence, residual and/or progression was more common. Patients submitted to partial removal plus XRT were also living, but with the neoplasm.

The **evidence-based systematic review** [16] about **MPE** revealed that XRT after surgery was very important to reduce significantly the tumor recurrence rate, even after GTR of the neoplasm.

The studies are currently supporting the role of **routine postoperative radiotherapy** to potentially reduce the recurrence/progression of the tumor in patients **operated for myxopapillary ependymoma**, even in patients who underwent gross-total resection [1, 16, 29, 41, 63].

CONCLUSION

This chapter reviewed and discussed the most relevant aspects of **intramedullary and myxopapillary ependymomas**, including the main clinical symptoms and their neuroradiological features, provided a description of modern surgical techniques and adjuvant therapy, and discussed the postoperative results and outcomes on the basis of University of Wisconsin series and the evidence-based systematic review of the literature.

This review was also mainly based on **level IV** of **medical evidence, recommendation grade C**, supporting:

- **Early diagnosis** and **better preoperative neurological status** can correlate with a better postoperative neurological **outcome** in patients treated with **intraspinal ependymoma**;
- **Gross total resection** in patients with **intraspinal ependymoma**, especially when such a resection can be accomplished without major morbidity;
- **Postoperative radiotherapy** to reduce the recurrence/progression of the tumor in patients with **intraspinal ependymoma** submitted to **incomplete resection;**
- **Routine postoperative radiotherapy** to potentially reduce the recurrence/progression of the tumor in patients **operated** for **myxopapillary ependymoma**, even in patients who underwent gross-total resection.

Intraspinal ependymoma is not as "benign" as proposed by its histology, but has a high potential of recurrence and/or progression. Although there is still controversy regarding the best management of those patients, in this review, it could be noticed that **radiation therapy** is recommended as a **routine after surgery** for **myxopapillary ependymoma**.

ACKNOWLEDGMENTS

To my wife Rita, my children, Nicolas and Thomas, my parents, Antonio (*in memoriam*) and Zenina, and to my siblings, Marco, Marcio, Karla and Elvis, for the continuous support.

I am very thankful to my Mentor of my Postdoctoral fellow and my friend Dr Daniel Resnick, and to my Co-mentor, Dr Nathaniel Brooks, as well as to the Department of Neurosurgery of the University of Wisconsin.

I am very grateful to Dr Thomas Zdeblick and Dr Donlin Long, who were my Mentors of my Spine Fellow and my professional inspiration.

Funding

Figueiredo received fellowship support from CAPES (Ministry of Education, Brasilia, Brazil), to perform the Postdoctoral Research Fellowship at the University of Wisconsin about Intraspinal Ependymomas (2011-2012).

REFERENCES

[1] Akyurek, S; Chang, EL; Yu, TK; Little, D; Allen, PK; McCutcheon, I; Mahajan, A; Maor, MH; Woo, SY. Spinal myxopapillary ependymoma outcomes in patients treated with surgery and radiotherapy at M.D. Anderson Cancer Center. *J Neurooncol*, 2006, 80, 177-183.

[2] Awaya, H; Kaneko, M; Amatya, VJ; Takeshima, Y; Oka, S; Inai, K. Myxopapillary ependymoma with anaplastic features. *Pathol Int*, 2003, 53, 700-703.

[3] Barone, BM; Elvidge, AR. Ependymomas: A clinical survey. *J Neurosurg*, 1970, 33, 428-438.

[4] Bono, CM; Watters, WC 3rd; Heggeness, MH; Resnick, DK; Shaffer, WO; Baisden, J; Ben-Galim, P; Easa, JE; Fernand, R; Lamer, T; Matz, PG; Mendel, RC; Patel, RK; Reitman, CA; Toton, JF. An evidence-based clinical guideline for the use of antithrombotic therapies in spine surgery. *Spine J*, 2009, 9, 1046-1051.

[5] Central Brain Tumor Registry of the United States (CBTRUS): Statistical report: Primary brain tumor in the United States, 2000-2004. (http://www.cbtrus.org/reports/ 2007-2008/2007report.pdf (Accessed October 10, 2011).

[6] Cervoni, L; Celli, P; Cantore, G; Fortuna, A. Intradural tumors of the cauda equina: a single institution review of clinical characteristics. *Clin Neurol Neurosurg*, 1995, 97, 8–12.

[7] Chamberlain, MC. Ependymomas. *Curr Neurolol Neurosci*, 2003, Rep 3, 193-199.

[8] Chamberlain, MC; Tredway, TL. Adult primary intradural spinal cord tumors: a review. *Curr Neurolol Neurosci Rep*, 2011, 11, 320-328.

[9] Chiang, HY; Herwaldt, LA; Blevins, AE; Cho, E; Schweizer, ML. Effectiveness of local vancomycin powder to decrease surgical site infections. *Spine J*, 2014, 14, 397-407.

[10] Christine, L; Hammer, San Jay; Yadla, James; Harrop, S. Techniques for Intradural Tumor Resection. In: Zdeblick TA, Albert T, eds. The Spine, Philadelphia: *Lippincott Williams and Wilkins*, 2014, 385-396.

[11] Clauss, EB; Abdel-Wahab, M; Burger, PC; Engelhard, HH; Ellison, DW; Gaiano, N; Gutmann, DH; Heck, DA; Holland, EC; Jallo, GI; Kruchko, C; Kun, LE; Maria, BL; Rumboldt, Z; Seminara, D; Spinella, GM; Stophel, L; Wechsler-Reya, R; Wrensch, M; Gilbertson, RJ. Defining future directions in spinal cord tumor research. Proceedings from the National Institutes of Health workshop. *J Neurosurg Spine*, 2010, 12, 117-121.

[12] Ellis, JA; Canoll, P; McCormick, PC. 2nd; Feldstein, NA; Anderson, RC; Kaiser, MG; McCormick, PC; Bruce, JN; Ogden, AT. Platelet-derived growth factor receptor(PDGFR) expression in primary spinal cord gliomas. *J Neurooncol*, 2012, 106, 235-242.

[13] Engelhard, HH; Villano, JL; Porter, KR; Stewart, AK; Barua, M; Barker, FG; et al. Clinical presentation, histology, and treatment in 430 patients with primary tumors of the spinal cord, spinal meninges, or cauda equine. *J Neurosurg Spine*, 2010, 13, 67-77.

[14] Fasset, DR; Schmidt, MH. Lumbosacral ependymomas: a review of the management of the intradural and extradural tumors. *Neurosurg Focus*, 2003,15, 1-5.

[15] Figueiredo, N; Brooks, N; Hanna, A; Baskaya, M; Trost, G; Resnick, D. Intraspinal ependymomas: case series study of myxopapillary and intramedullary ependymomas. *Chirurgia*, 2013, 26, 101-110.

[16] Figueiredo, N; Brooks, N; Resnick, D. Evidence-based review and guidelines for the management of myxopapillary and intramedullary ependymoma. *Journal of Neurosurgical Sciences*, 2013, 57, 327-341.

[17] Gezen, F; Kahraman, S; Canakei, Z; Beduk, A. Review of 36 cases of spinal cord meningioma. *Spine*, 2000, 25, 727-731.

[18] Gomez, DR. High failure rate in spinal ependymomas with long-term follow-up. *Neuro-Oncology*, 2005, 7, 254–259.

[19] Grahame-Smith, D. Evidence based medicine: Socratic dissent. *BMJ*, 1995,29, 1126-1127.

[20] Helseth, A; Mork, SJ. Primary intraspinal neoplasms in Norway, 1955 to 1986. A population-based survey of 467 patients. *J Neurosurg*, 1989, 71, 842–845.

[21] Hida, K. Intramedullary spinal cord tumors. In: The textbook of spinal surgery. Bridwell K, DeWald RL, eds. Philadelphia: *Lippincott Williams and Wilkins*, 2011, 1520-1534.

[22] Kaiser, MG; Eck, JC; Groff, MW; Watters, WC 3rd; Dailey, AT; Resnick, DK; Choudhri, TF; Sharan, A; Wang, JC; Mummaneni, PV; Dhall, SS; Ghogawala, Z. Guidelines for the performance of fusion procedures for degenerative disease of the lumbar spine. *J Neurosurg: Spine*, 2014, 21, 2-16.

[23] Khan, NR; Thompson, CJ; DeCuypere, M; Angotti, JM; Kalobwe, E; Muhlbauer, MS; Camillo, FX; Klimo, P Jr. A meta-analysis of spinal surgical site infection and vancomycin powder. *J Neurosurg Spine*, 2014, 21, 974-983.

[24] Kim, DH; Kim, JH, Choi, SH; Sohn, CH; Yun, TJ, Kim, CH, Chang, KH. Differentiation between Intramedullary spinal ependymoma and astrocytoma: Comparative MRI analysis. *Clinical Radiology*, 2014, 69, 29-35.

[25] Klekamp, J; Samii, M. Surgery of Spinal Tumors: Intramedullary Tumors. Berlin: Springer-Verlag, 2007, 20-141.

[26] Klekamp, J; Samii, M. Surgery of Spinal Tumors: Extramedullary Tumors. Berlin: Springer-Verlag, 2007, 143-320.

[27] Koeller, KK; Rosenblum, RS; Morrison, AL. Neoplasms of the spinal cord and filum terminale: radiologic-pathologic correlation. *RadioGraphics*, 2000, 20, 1721-1749.

[28] Kucia, EJ; Bambakidis, NC; Chang, SW; Spetzler, RF. Surgical technique and outcomes in the treatment of spinal cord ependymomas: part I: intramedullary ependymoma. *Operative Neurosurgery*, 2011, 68, 57-63.

[29] Kucia, EJ; Maughan, PH; Kakarla, UK; Bambakidis, NC; Spetzler, RF. Surgical technique and outcomes in the treatment of spinal cord ependymomas, part II: myxopapillary ependymoma. *Operative Neurosurgery*, 2011, 68, 90-94.

[30] Louis, DN; Ohgaki, H; Wiestler, OD; Cavence, WK; Burger, PC; Jouvet, A; Scheithauer, BW; Kleihues, P. The 2007 WHO classification of tumours of the central nervous system. *Acta Neuropathol*, 2007, 114, 97-109.

[31] Manzano, G; Green, BA; Vanni, S; Levi, AD. Contemporary management of adult intramedullary spinal tumors: pathology and neurological outcomes related to surgical resection. *Spinal Cord*, 2008, 46, 540-546.
[32] Marks, JE; Adler, SJ. A comparative study of ependymomas by site of origin. *Int J Radiat Oncol Biol Phys*, 1982, 8, 37-43.
[33] Matsuyama, Y; Sakai, Y; Katayama, Y; Imagama, S; Ito, Z; Wakao, N; Sato, K; Kamiya, M; Yukawa, Y; Kanemura, T; Yanase, M; Ishiguro, N. Surgical results of intramedullary spinal cord tumor with spinal cord monitoring to guide extent of resection. *J Neurosurg Spine*, 2009, 10, 404-413.
[34] McCormick, PC; Stein, BM. Intramedullary tumors in adults. *Neurosurg Clin N Am*, 1990, 1, 609–630.
[35] McCormick, PC; Torres, R; Post, KD; Stein, BM. Intramedullary ependymoma of the spinal cord. *J Neurosurg*, 1990, 72, 523–532.
[36] McGirt, MJ; Garces-Ambrossi, GL; Parker, SL; Sciubba, DM; Bydon, A; Wolinksy, JP; Gokaslan, ZL; Jallo, G; Witham, TF. Short-term Progressive Spinal Deformity Following Laminoplasty Versus Laminectomy for Resection of Intradural Spinal Tumors: Analysis of 238 Patients. *Neurosurgery*, 2010, 66, 1005-1012.
[37] McGuire, CS; Sainani, KL; Fisher, PG. Incidence patterns for ependymoma: a surveillance, epidemiology, and end results study. *J Neurosurg*, 2009, 110, 725–729.
[38] McLaughlin, MP; Buatti, JM; Marcua, RB; Jr. Maria, BL; Mickle, PJ; Kedar, A. Outcome after radiotherapy of primary spinal cord glial tumors. *Radiat Oncol Invest*, 1998, 6, 276-280.
[39] Miyazawa, N; Hida, K; Iwasaki, Y; Koyanagi, I; Abe, H. MRI at 1.5 T of intramedullary ependymoma and classification of pattern of contrast enhancement. *Neuroradiology*, 2000, 42, 828-832.
[40] Montano, NG; Cioni, B; Lucantoni, C; Della Pepa, GM; Meglio, M; Papacci, F. The role of laminoplasty in preventing spinal deformity in adult patients submitted to resection of an intradural spinal tumor. Case series and literature review. *Clin Neurol Neurosurg*, 2014, 125, 69-74.
[41] Nakamura, M; Ishii, K; Watanabe, K; Tsuji, T; Matsumoto, M; Toyama, Y; Chiba, K. Long-term surgical outcomes for myxopapillary ependymomas of the cauda equina. *Spine*, 2009, 34, E756-760.
[42] Nittner, K. Spinal meningiomas, neurinomas and neurofibromas, and hourglass tumours. In: Vinken, PH; Bruyn, GW, eds. Handbook of Clinical Neurology. Elsevier: New York, 1976, 177-322.
[43] Oh, MC; Ivan, ME; Sun, MZ; Kaur, G; Safaee, M; Kim, JM; Sayegh, ET; Aranda, D; Parsa, AT. Adjuvant radiotherapy delays recurrence following subtotal resection of spinal cord ependymomas. *Neuro Oncol*, 2013, 15, 208-215.
[44] Parsa, AT; Chi, JH; Acosta, FL; Ames, CP; McCormick, PC. Intramedullary Spinal Cord Tumors: Molecular insights and Surgical Innovation. *Clinical Neurosurgery*, 2005, 52, 49-50.
[45] Parsa, AT; Lee, J; Parney, IF; Weinstein, P; McCormick, PC; Ames, C. Spinal cord and intradural extraparenchyma spinal tumors: current best care practices and strategies. *J Neurooncol*, 2004, 69, 291-318.
[46] Pica, A; Miller, R; Villa, S; Kadish, SP; Anacak, Y; Abusaris, H; Ozyigit, G; Baumert, BG; Zaucha, R; Haller, G; Weber, DC. The results of surgery, with or without

radiotherapy, for primary spinal myxopapillary ependymoma: a retrospective study from the Rare Cancer Network. *Int J Radiation Oncology Biol Phys*, 2009, 74, 1114-1120.

[47] Quigley, DG; Farooqi, N; Pigott, TJD; Findlay, G; Pillay, R; Buxton, N; Jenkinson, MD. Outcome predictors in the management of spinal cord ependymoma. *Eur Spine J*, 2007, 16, 399-404.

[48] Rawlings, CE; Giangaspero, F; Burger, PC; Bullard, DE. Ependymomas: a clinicopathologic study. *Surg Neurol*, 1988, 29, 271–281.

[49] Rhines, LD; Groves, MD. Tumors of the spinal cord and intradural space. DeMonte, F; Gilbert, MR; Mahajan, A; McCutcheon, IE, eds., Tumors of the Brain and Spine. M.D. Anderson Cancer Care Series. New York: Springer, 2007, 295-328.

[50] Sackett, DL; Rosenberg, WM; Gray, JA; Haynes, RB; Richardson, WS. Evidence based medicine: what it is and what it isn't. *BMJ*, 1996, 312, 71–72.

[51] Sala, F; Bricolo, A; Faccioli, F; Lanteri, P; Gerosa, M. Surgery for intramedullary spinal cord tumors: the role of intraoperative (neurophysiological) monitoring. *Eur Spine J*, 2007, 16 Suppl 2, S130-139.

[52] Schellinger, KA; Propp, JM; Villano, JL; McCarthy, BJ. Descriptive epidemiology of primary spinal cord tumors. *J Neurooncol*, 2008, 87, 173-179, 2008.

[53] Schild, SE; Nisi, K; Scheithauer, BW; Wong, WW; Lyons, MK; Schomberg, PJ; Shaw, EG. The results of radiotherapy for ependymomas: the Mayo clinic experience. *Int J Radiation Oncology Biol Phys*, 1998, 42, 953-958.

[54] Schwartz, TH; McCormick, PC. Intramedullary ependymomas: clinical presentation, surgical treatment strategies and prognosis. *J Neurooncol*, 2000, 41, 211-218.

[55] Schweitzer, J; Batzdorf, U. Ependymoma of the cauda equina region: diagnosis, treatment, and outcome in 15 patients. *Neurosurgery*, 1992, 30, 202-207.

[56] Sciubba, DM; Liang, D; Kothbauer, KF; Noggle, JC; Jallo, GI. The evolution of intramedullary spinal cord tumor surgery. *Neurosurgery*, 2009, 65, 84-92.

[57] Shaffer, WO; Baisden, JL; Fernand, R; Matz, PG.North American Spine Society. An evidence-based clinical guideline for antibiotic prophylaxis in spine surgery.*Spine J*, 2013, 13, 1387-1392.

[58] Shirato, H; Kamada, T; Hida, K; Koyanagi, I; Iwasaki, Y; Miyasaka, K; Abe, H. The role of radiotherapy in the management of spinal cord glioma. *Int J Radiat Oncol Biol Phys*, 1995, 33, 323-328.

[59] Sonneland, PRL; Scheithauer, BW; Onofrio, BM. Myxopapillary ependymoma: A clinicopathologic and immunocytochemical study of 77 cases. *Cancer*, 1985, 56, 883-893.

[60] Struffert, T; Grunwald, I; Roth, C; Reith, W. Spinal intradural e tumore. *Radiologe*, 2004, 44, 1211–1228.

[61] Sun, B; Wang, C; Wang, J; Liu, A. MRI features of intramedullary spinal cord ependymomas. *J Neuroimaging*, 2003, 13, 346–351.

[62] Szelényi, A; Heukamp, C; Seifert, V; Marquardt, GS. 100B, intraoperative neuromonitoring findings and their relation to clinical outcome in surgically treated intradural spinal lesions. *Acta Neurochir (Wien)*, 2014, 156, 733-739.

[63] Tsai, CJ; Wang, Y; Allen, PK; Mahajan, A; McCutcheon, IE; Rao, G; Rhines, LD; Tatsui, CE; Armstrong, TS; Maor, MH; Chang, EL; Brown, PD; Li, J. Outcomes after surgery and radiotherapy for spinal myxopapillary ependymoma: update of the MD Anderson Cancer Center experience. *Neurosurgery*, 2014, 75, 205-214.

[64] Tseng, JH; Tseng, MY. Survival analysis of 459 adult patients with primary spinal cancer in England and Wales: a population-based study. *Surg Neurol*, 2007, 67, 53–58.
[65] Yagi, T; Ohata, K; Haque, M; Hakuba, A. Intramedullary spinal cord tumour associated with neurofibromatosis type 1. *Acta Neurochir (Wien)*, 1997, 139, 1055–1060.
[66] Yanni, DS; Ulbakatan, S; Deletius, V; Barrenehea, IJ; Sen, C; Perin, NI. Utility of neurophysiological monitoring using dorsal column mapping in intramedullary spinal cord surgery. *J Neurosurg Spine*, 2010, 12, 623-628.
[67] Yonekawa, Y; Marugg, R. Intradural Tumors. In: Boos, N; Aebi, M, eds. Berlin: Springer-Verlag. *Spinal Disorders: Fundamental of Diagnosis and Treatment*, 2008, 997-1019.
[68] Wen, BC; Hussey, DH; Hitchon, PW; Schelper, RL; Vigliotti, AP; Doornbos, JF; VanGilder, JC. The role of radiation therapy in the management of ependymomas of the spinal cord. *Int J Radiat Oncol Biol Phys*, 1991, 20, 781-786.
[69] Wippold, FJ; Smirniotopoulos, JC; Moran, CJ; Suojanen, JN; Volmer, DG. MR imaging of myxopapillary ependymoma: findings and value to determine extent of tumor and its relation to intraspinal structures. *Am J Roentgenol*, 1995, 165, 1263-1267.

In: Ependymomas
Editor: Raquel Fowler

ISBN: 978-1-63484-405-5

Chapter 5

Ependymomas Arising in the Setting of Hereditary Tumor Syndromes

Rachel A. Wilson*[1], *BA, Brigid E. Prayson*[1], *BA, and Richard A. Prayson*[2,*], *MD, MEd
[1]John Carroll University and
[2]Department of Anatomic Pathology, Cleveland Clinic,
Cleveland, OH, US

Abstract

The vast majority of ependymal neoplasms appear to arise in a sporadic fashion. There are, however, subsets of these neoplasms that are known to be associated with hereditary tumor syndromes or neurocutaneous disorders. The most recognized of these associations is the predisposition of Neurofibromatosis Type II (NF2) patients toward the development of certain nervous system tumors including ependymomas, vestibular and schwannomas, and meningiomas. NF2 gene mutations (chromosome 22q12.2) are well-recognized features of these patients and their tumors. Less commonly, ependymomas have been reported in patients with MEN 1 syndrome, which is characterized by the development of multiple endocrine neoplasms. The MEN 1 gene (chromosome 11q13) is involved in allelic losses and rearrangements in ependymomas. Ependymomas have also been described rarely in patients with Turcot syndrome (MSH2 gene on chromosome 2p22-p21). Anecdotal cases of ependymoma have also been described in association with disorders such as Li-Fraumeni syndrome, Neurofibromatosis Type I, Cowden syndrome, von Hippel-Lindau syndrome and Tuberous Sclerosis. This chapter reviews the literature on ependymal neoplasms arising in the setting of hereditary tumor syndromes.

[*] Correspondence: Richard Prayson, MD, Med, Department of Anatomic Pathology, L25, Cleveland Clinic, 9500 Euclid Avenue, Cleveland, OH 44195 USA, Phone: 216-444-8805, FAX: 216-445-6967, Email: praysor@ccf.org.

INTRODUCTION

Ependymomas are relatively uncommon neoplasms of the brain and spinal cord in adults, but they account for approximately 10% of all intracranial tumors of childhood and as much as 30% of intracranial tumors in some series of children less than 3 years of age [1]. Tumors are generally graded as low grade (WHO grade II) and anaplastic (WHO grade III) based on the presence or absence of certain histologic parameters including mitoses, cellularity, vascular proliferative changes and necrosis [2]. Higher-grade lesions are well accepted to carry a worse prognosis [1, 3]. Low grade variants, WHO grade I, namely subependymoma and myxopapillary ependymoma, are well established entities. Clinical presentations are location dependent and may include signs and symptoms related to hydrocephalus and increased intracranial pressure (headaches, nausea, vomiting, and dizziness). Cerebellar tumors may present with ataxia, dizziness, paresis, and visual disturbances. Supratentorial lesions may present with seizures, focal neurological deficits and intracranial hypertension. Spinal tumors typically manifest with motor and sensory deficits. Treatment includes surgical excision, if possible, accompanied variously by radiotherapy and chemotherapy.

The majority of ependymal neoplasms appear to arise in a sporadic fashion. However, there are small subsets of cases that appear to arise as part of a hereditary tumor syndrome (neurocutaneous disorder, phakomatosis). This review is focused on examining these subsets of ependymal tumors.

NEUROFIBROMATOSIS TYPE II

Neurofibromatosis Type II (NF2) is an autosomal dominant disorder that predisposes individuals to develop schwannomas of the eighth cranial nerve (commonly bilateral), schwannomas of other cranial and peripheral nerves, meningiomas, ependymomas, and rarely astrocytomas (Figures 1 and 2). NF2 is associated with mutations in the gene encoding Neurofibromin 2; the gene is located on chromosome 22q12.2 and provides instructions for the development of tumor suppressor protein merlin (schwannomin) [4-6]. Since Neurofibromin 2 is the only gene in which a mutation is known to cause NF2, genetic testing may be done looking for a mutation [7]. Birth incidence is significantly higher than diagnostic prevalence at 1 in 33,000-40,000 [8].

Symptom onset in NF2 generally occurs between 18 and 24 years of age, yet reports have indicated an onset range of birth to 70 years of age [8]. Since NF2 is usually viewed as an adult-onset disease, frequent misdiagnosis may occur in children. Tumors of the skin and ocular findings may be the first indicators of the disease [7, 9]. A majority of patients present with bilateral vestibular schwannomas, an NF2 hallmark, by the age of 30 years. Another two-thirds will develop spinal tumors with 5-33% presenting with intramedullary tumors, including astrocytomas and ependymomas. Furthermore, nearly half of those with NF2 have meningiomas (lifetime risk of 80%). Spinal meningiomas may occur, although most are intracranial. In addition, a third of individuals will present with decreased visual acuity. Mononeuropathy, particularly affecting the facial nerve, has also been noted as a recognizable feature [8].

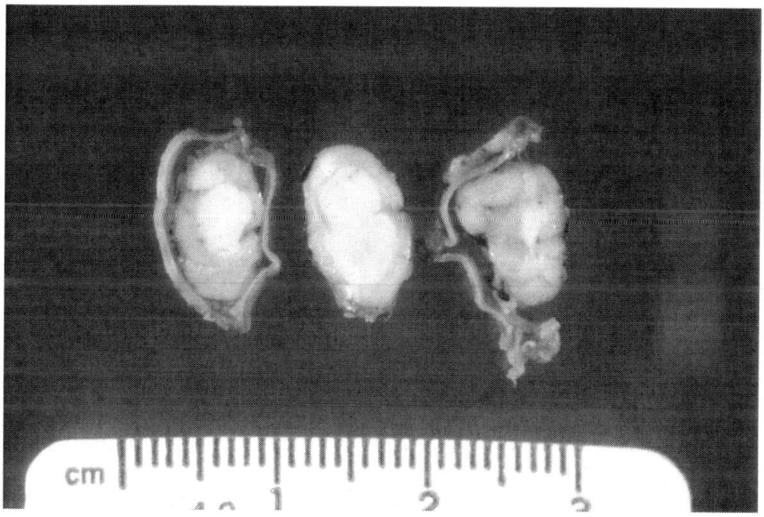

Figure 1. Gross appearance at autopsy in a 33-year-old woman with Neurofibromatosis Type II showing an intramedullary mass involving the thoracic spinal cord.

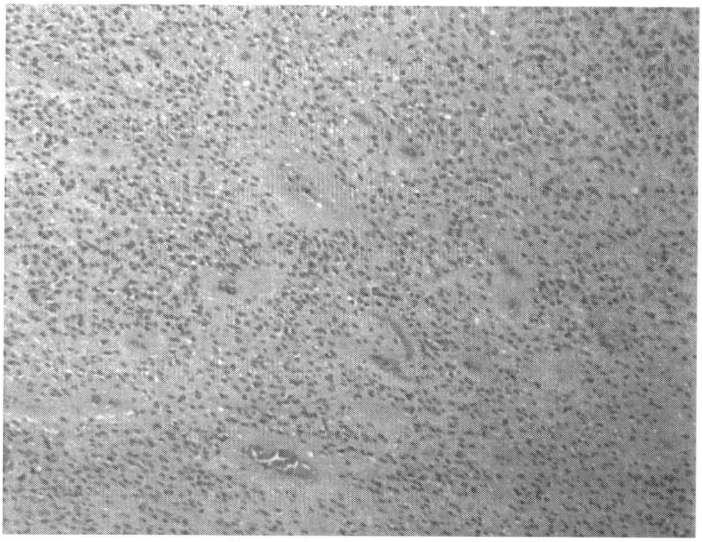

Figure 2. A photograph of the intramedullary mass seen in Figure 1 showed a low grade ependymoma, WHO grade II, marked by the presence of prominent perivascular pseudorosette formations (hematoxylin and eosin, original magnification 200X).

NF2 manifests differently in affected individuals based on varying tumor location, size and number. Symptoms may include balance dysfunction, ophthalmic features, such as cataracts and vision changes, tinnitus, unilateral hearing loss, café-au-lait spots, headaches, and weakness of the face. Patient lifespan is decreased as a result of ongoing complications. Surgical removal of tumors remains the primary course of treatment for symptomatic individuals. It is believed that surveillance is reasonable for asymptomatic ependymomas in the setting of NF2 [10].

A clinical diagnosis may be made in individuals who meet one of the following criteria: 1) bilateral vestibular schwannomas; 2) a first-degree relative with NF2 and unilateral vestibular schwannoma or two of the following lesions including meningioma, schwannoma, glioma, neurofibroma, posterior subcapsular lenticular opacities; 3) a unilateral vestibular schwannoma and any two of the following: meningioma, schwannoma, glioma, neurofibroma, posterior subcapsular lenticular opacities; or 4) multiple meningiomas and unilateral vestibular schwannoma or any two of the following: schwannoma, glioma, neurofibroma, and cataract [8].

In a large series, Plotkin et al. reported on 55 NF2 patients who had imaging findings consistent with ependymomas between 1994 and 2007 [10]. In three of the patients, ependymomas were the initial presentation of NF2. Of the 55 patients, 29 patients had clinically unaffected parents, with 26 having affected relatives. A total of 121 ependymomas were identified through magnetic resonance imaging (MRI); 58% of patients had multiple ependymomas. The most common site of involvement was cervical spine and cerviocomedullary junction (85.5% of patients), followed by the thoracic spine (61.9% of patients) and lumbar spine (7.3% of patients). Most patients were asymptomatic and did not require surgical intervention; however, 11 individuals did require surgery after symptomatic progression. Of these 11 tumors, nine were classified as WHO grade II, including a single tumor containing some anaplastic features, one tumor was classified as WHO grade I and a biopsy of another demonstrated atypical glial cells without a definitive pathological diagnosis. Of those who were symptomatic, eight had motor and sensory loss, five had back and leg pain, and two presented with gait disturbances. The median age of diagnosis was 21 years.

Hagel et al. reported similar symptoms after a re-evaluation of 12 spinal gliomas in NF2 patients, 10 of which were previously diagnosed as ependymomas and two as astrocytomas [11]. Gait abnormality was the most common symptom with several patients presenting with neck, arm and back pain. Immunohistochemistry results typically showed dot-like and ring-shaped cytoplasmic positivity for epithelial membrane antigen (EMA). Most tumors arose in the cervical region of the spine, with rare cases arising in the thoracic spine. All tumors were classified as WHO grade II.

While tanycytic ependymomas are rare, this subtype has been reported in NF2 [12-13]. Lim et al. reported a 16-year-old girl who presented with gait disturbance and a palpable neck mass, which was present for two years [12]. Neurological examination revealed left elbow extension weakness. No sensory disturbance or hearing loss was noted. A MRI revealed multiple intradural, intramedullary and extramedullary masses throughout the spinal canal with bilateral vestibular schwannomas and multiple masses in the left supraclavicular area, axilla, and right cavernous sinus. Surgical removal was the course of treatment for the intramedullary mass and a diagnosis of tanycytic ependymoma rendered. The tumor was marked by elongated spindle-shaped cells that were immunopositive for S-100 protein, epithelial membrane antigen, and glial fibrillary acidic protein [12]. Symptoms improved and a MRI indicated there was no evidence of tumor enlargement after two years. Ueki et al. described a tanycytic ependymoma in an 18-year-old female with NF2 who had bilateral acoustic tumors and a meningioma at the planum sphenoidale [13]. This individual presented with an intramedullary mass at the T-1 level, which was eventually removed surgically. Histological examination showed that the tumor consisted of elongated spindle shaped cells, which were immunopositive for S-100 protein and glial fibrillary and acidic protein. Ultrastructural examination showed microvilli-lined lamina and prominent intercellular junctions, characteristic ependymal tumors [13].

In 2011, Aguilera et al. reported two cases of cervicomedullary tumors in patients with NF2 [4]. The first patient was treated with subtotal resection after histological confirmation of ependymoma. The patient had no progression after 11 months. The second patient was observed for several years without treatment for a cervicomedullary tumor and did not present with any clinical symptoms. Another 21 cases of ependymoma were mentioned in the literature review in this paper (14 males and 7 females); the spine was the most common location reported for 12 patients (57%). In the infratentorial location, the median age was 12 years, and for spinal ependymomas the median age was 15 years. Surgical removal of tumors was the most common treatment approach. Of the 17 patients who underwent surgical treatment, 5 patients had a gross total resection (GTR) and 11 patients had subtotal resection (STR). No surgical procedure was specified for one of the patients. Eight of nine patients with infratentorial ependymomas underwent STR and one patient did not undergo surgery. For spinal ependymomas, five patients had GTR, four had STR and in three patients the extent of tumor resection was not reported. Pathology revealed ependymomas, (not further specified) in 13, subependymomas in two, tanycytic ependymomas in three, one low-grade ependymoma and one malignant ependymoma. No treatment with radiation was reported. Among patients with infratentorial tumors, five were alive at last known follow-up and four were deceased. Among these with spinal tumors, 11 are alive and one is deceased. No correlation between location and survival rate was seen.

Nine patients with neurofibromatosis and intramedullary spinal cord tumors were mentioned in a report that after histological examination concluded five ependymomas, three astrocytomas and one intramedullary schwannoma [14]. The intramedullary ependymomas were almost all associated with NF2 and astrocytomas with NF1 individuals. In one patient with an ependymoma, the NF type was unknown.

NEUROFIBROMATOSIS TYPE I

Neurofibromatosis Type I (NF1) is a multisystem, autosomal dominant genetic disorder of the nervous system characterized by growth and development abnormalities of nerve cell tissues. Common manifestations of NF1 include neurofibromas, café-au-lait spots, optic gliomas, Lisch nodules, scoliosis, bone overgrowth, and freckling in areas that lack sun exposure. Nearly 10% of individuals with NF1 present with malignant peripheral nerve sheath tumors, which are the most common malignant tumor associated with this syndrome [15]. The overall incidence is 1 in 3,000 individuals, making NF1 one of the most common inherited disorders [15].

Nearly half of those with NF1 inherit the disorder from a parent. The remaining half of patients will have a gene mutation in Neurofibromin 1, also known as the NF1 gene, located on chromosome 17q11.2 [16]. Mutations within the gene most likely contribute to uncontrolled cell growth and proliferation due to the gene either preventing a protein from being made or causing the protein to be made incorrectly [15].

Clinical diagnosis requires two out of seven of the following criterion to be identified: six or more café-au-lait macules (>0.5 cm in children or >1.5 cm in adults), two or more cutaneous/subcutaneous neurofibromas or one plexiform neurofibroma, axillary or groin freckling (>2 freckles), optic pathway gliomas, 2 or more Lisch nodules (iris hamartomas) typically identified through slit lamp examination, sphenoid dysplasia or typical long-bone abnormalities such as pseudarthrosis, and a first-degree relative with NF1 [17]. NF1 cannot be prevented; however, proper management of symptoms is the preferred course of treatment.

Although uncommon, ependymomas have been reported in NF1. Most recently, Hongwei et al. presented a case of a cervical spinal cord ependymoma (grade II) arising in a 49-year-old woman with NF1 [16]. She was admitted after experiencing numbness in her fingers that progressed above the navel for six months. She had a previous history of malignant neurofibromas, café-au-lait spots, axillary and groin freckles, cutaneous neurofibromas, and plexiform neurofibromas. A family history of NF1 was noted. A MRI revealed a relatively demarcated, heterogeneously enhancing mass lesion accompanied by edema at the C5-7 level, a left-sided T11 spinous process heterogeneously enhancing mass in the soft tissue, intervertebral disk hernia at the L2-5 level, and a widespread enhancing lesion at the T11-L5 level. A posterior laminectomy was performed from C5-7 after determination of location by ultrasonography and the tumor was removed. One year post-operatively, neurological symptoms remained diminished.

Riffaud et al. reported four cases of hemispheric cerebral glioma in children with NF1, in which two of the tumors were ependymomas [18]. Riffaud et al. describe a 7-year-old boy with an isolated asymptomatic left temporal lesion that was detected after routine magnetic resonance imaging examination. A history of NF1 was noted in the family. The child presented with café-au-lait spots. After a normal neurological examination, radiological and clinical follow-up was suggested. A MRI showed an increase in lesion size two years later, in which the lesion was removed via a left temporal craniotomy. A benign ependymoma (grade II) was revealed during a histopathological examination. No additional treatment was given after the removal and the patient had no recurrence.

Riffaud et al. also described a 12-year-old girl with an isolated, asymptomatic left temporal lesion that was also detected during a routine MRI examination [18]. Café-au-lait spots were also present as well as a family history of NF1. A neurological exam was normal. After eight months of no treatment, the girl presented with headaches and dyslexia; a MRI showed a great increase in lesion size. A left temporo-parietal craniotomy was performed to remove the lesion. Partial tonic-clonic seizures of the right side of the body occurred postoperatively and were resolved with medication. Histopathological examination revealed a malignant ependymoma (grade III). Radiotherapy was administered. Three months later, a recurrence involving the upper cervical spinal cord and brain stem was seen. The girl was diagnosed with meningeal spread, which was confirmed by histopathological analysis of cerebrospinal fluid. The patient began chemotherapy and subsequently passed away five months later due to cachexia.

Sharma et al. reported a 55-year-old man with NF1 who presented with hypertension and recurrent falls [19]. Poor coordination, impaired joint position, and a positive Romberg's test were noted. No abnormal neurological findings were mentioned. An intramedullary spine lesion at the T8-L1 level was observed on MRI and subsequently resected. A diagnosis of low-grade ependymoma was rendered.

MULTIPLE ENDOCRINE NEOPLASIA TYPE I

Multiple Endocrine Neoplasia (MEN) Type I or Wermer Syndrome represents an autosomal dominant condition marked by mutations in the MEN1 gene on chromosome 11q13 [20-21]. Mutations have been reported in up to 80-90% of familial cases using sequence analysis [20].

Most commonly, the syndrome is associated with the development of parathyroid tumors (usually manifesting with hypercalcemia), pituitary adenomas (most commonly prolactinomas) and well differentiated endocrine tumors of the gastro-entero-pancreatic tract. Diagnostic criteria include the presence of two out of these three main endocrine tumor types. Familial MEN1 syndrome is defined in an individual who has MEN1 syndrome with either one first degree relative with one or more of these endocrine neoplasms or single organ involvement and a MEN1 germline pathogenic variant. Combinations of over 20 different endocrine and nonendocrine related tumors have been variously described in this syndrome making the development of a straightforward, all-encompassing definition complicated. Among the other tumors that have been described as being associated with this syndrome include carcinoid tumors, adrenocortical tumors, facial angiofibromas, collagenomas, lipomas and leiomyomas [22].

Tumors of the central nervous system arising in the setting of MEN1 are unusual and have included cases of meningioma and ependymoma. Ashgarian et al. in a prospective study of 74 MEN 1 patients, noted meningiomas in six patients (8%) [23]. The meningiomas were single lesions arising late in the disease course (mean age 51 years). The tumors were asymptomatic and the majority of them showed no growth.

Only anecdotal cases of ependymomas arising in the setting of MEN I have been described in the literature [24-27]. In 1996, Kato et al. reported on a 51-year-old male who presented with gait disturbance and hypoesthesia below the level of his chest [24]. The family history was significant for insulinoma in his two sons and paternal cousin. Imaging studies of the spine (magnetic resonance imaging) revealed an intramedullary lesion at the cervico-thoracic level (C5-T2) with associated syringomyelia. The patient underwent gross total resection of the tumor which was diagnosed as a "benign ependymoma". He was subsequently diagnosed with parathyroid hyperplasia and a pituitary microadenoma.

Giraud and colleagues briefly mentioned a woman in kindred who was diagnosed with hyperparathyroidism at age 26 years [25]. Three years later, she developed hypoesthesia and weakness in the left leg. A 9 cm spinal cord mass between the eighth and tenth vertebrae with associated syrinx was discovered. The mass was excised and diagnosed as a papillary ependymoma grade II.

In a letter to the editor, Al-Salameh and coworkers described a 44-year-old woman, with a previous history of multiple insulinomas of the pancreas and parathyroid adenoma who presented with memory loss and disorientation to space and time [26]. A MRI study showed a 4 cm mass in the pineal gland region with associated hydrocephaly. The tumor was resected and a diagnosis of grade II ependymoma was rendered. Tumor recurrence was diagnosed 14 months later and the resection showed an ependymoma with "high mitotic activity and a higher degree of proliferation (higher value of MIB-1, a cell proliferation marker) in comparison with the initial ependymoma". The patient expired 7 months later.

In 2013, a case report of a tanycytic ependymoma arising in the filum terminale region was published [27]. The patient was a 53-year-old male who presented with complaints of nocturnal pain in the lower back accompanied by perianal numbness and intermittent claudication. A MRI study identified an intradural, enhancing mass at the level of T12-L2. The tumor was diagnosed as a WHO grade II neoplasm. The patient showed no evidence of tumor recurrence 32 months postoperatively on MRI imaging.

Of anecdotal interest is a case report by Spaulding et al. reporting an ependymoma and carcinoid tumor associated with an ovarian mature cystic teratoma in a woman with MEN 1 [28]. The tumor was discovered in a 51-year-old woman on a computed tomographic (CT) scan done as part of an evaluation for dysfunctional uterine bleeding. A solid nodule within the tumor had an area interpreted as resembling a "well differentiated ependymoma".

TURCOT SYNDROME

Glioma-polyposis syndrome or Turcot syndrome is a rare genetic disorder, which results in colonic polyposis and primary tumors of the central nervous system [29]. Two major types of genetic mutations differentiate or subclassify patients with Turcot syndrome either as having adenomatous polyposis coli (APC) or hereditary non-polyposis colon cancer (HNPCC).

The two most common brain tumors that arise in patients with Turcot syndrome include glioblastoma, more commonly seen in families with features of Lynch syndrome, and medulloblastoma, more commonly seen in families with features of familial adenomatous polyposis. Mutations in specific genes have been found to be associated with development of these syndromes and tumors. The MLH1 and the PMS2 genes have been implicated in families with glioblastoma and features of Lynch syndrome, while there seems to be an association within families with medulloblastoma and features of familial adenomatous polyposis with the APC gene [30].

Since Turcot syndrome is associated with tumor development in the central nervous system, it is not unexpected that patients with Turcot syndrome would develop ependymomas. A study on the molecular aspects of Turcot syndrome which analyzed data from 14 families found only one case of ependymoma in a patient with Turcot syndrome [31].

Only two known reports have described patients with Turcot syndrome having multiple ependymomas [32-33]. A 1997 case report described the medical history of a 21-year-old Hispanic woman who, at the age of 16-years-old, presented with limping and persistent pain in her right leg and ankle, which had lasted for several weeks [32]. She had a previous medical history of skull osteomas and hyper-pigmented spots on her right retina. At age 9 years, she underwent a partial colectomy for colonic polyposis; both her mother and brother had also undergone colon resection for polyposis. Beyond her immediate family, her maternal uncle and grandfather also had colonic polyposis, and ultimately died from colon cancer in their forties. MRI scans revealed a tumor in low sacral spinal canal and another tumor in her left cerebellopontine angle region. Both tumors were partially resected. The sacral tumor was diagnosed as a myxopapillary ependymoma and the cerebellar tumor was diagnosed as an anaplastic ependymoma. Additionally, she underwent radiation and chemotherapy. One year after surgery, tender subcutaneous masses were identified in the lumbosacral and thoracic region and she developed pain in the right lumbosacral paraspinal area coupled with weakness in the right leg and declining ability to walk. A MRI showed tumors in the right and left paraspinal regions; the lesions were grossly totally resected and identified as desmoids. Postoperatively, the patient's symptoms notably improved. Over the year, another large desmoid tumor developed in the patient's left upper thoracic paraspinal region. Evidence of ependymoma tumor recurrence was absent from additional MRI imaging. The authors reported this as being the first known instance of multiple CNS ependymomas in a patient with Turcot sundrome [32]. A subsequent report published in 1998 from the same institution as the aforementioned 1997 report, appeared to describe the same case [33].

Li-Fraumani Syndrome

Li-Fraumani syndrome (LFS) or Sarcoma, Breast, Leukemia and Adrenal Gland (SBLA) syndrome is a rare genetic tumor syndrome which most commonly results from germline mutations of the TP53 gene [34] and often gives rise to malignant neoplasms chiefly in young adults and children. Not all patients with LFS have the TP53 mutation, but instead may have mutations of related genes. Additionally, not all patients with mutations in the TP53 gene have LFS, and they may have other diseases including Diamond-Blackfan anemia, CHARGE syndrome and ATR-Seckel syndrome [35]. The CHEK2 tumor-suppressor gene has also been implicated in LFS, although whether it is directly related to LFS is presently uncertain [36]. The genetic profile accompanying LFS causes a predisposition to developing an assortment of malignancies [34].

There are several approaches to rendering a diagnosis of LFS. Typically, patients present with multiple tumors and a family history of tumors [37]. According to the National Institutes of Health, LFS is defined by all of the following: diagnosis of a proband with sarcoma before age 45 years old, possession of a first-degree relative with cancer before the age of 45 years old and having a first or second-degree relative with any cancer before the age of 45 years old or sarcoma at any age [38].

Only one known case report describes a LFS patient with ependymoma [34]. In a report describing the findings in a family with LFS, the father of the "index" patient was described as having an ependymoma. The index patient was an 11-year-old girl who had an anaplastic medulloblastoma. Her father presented with intervals of back pain in the lumbar region and a myxopapillary ependymoma (WHO grade I) was subtotally resected; the outcome of the patient was not indicated in the article. Due to the prevalence of tumors in the family medical history, with tumors arising in the CNS, an analysis of the TP53 genotype was performed. The index patient, her father and one of her two brothers was found to have a germline R248W TP53 missense mutation [34].

Cowden Syndrome

Cowden syndrome (CS) was first described in a 1963 case report [39] and has since been estimated to have a prevalence of greater than 1 in 200,000 [40]. CS results from a germline mutation of the PTEN gene [41-43]. This genetic alteration in the PTEN tumor suppressor gene (chromosome 10 tensin and phosphatase homologues) (10q23.3) [44] results in a predisposition to developing cancers in any of the three embryonic germ cell layers, as well as the development of noncancerous growths called hamartomas. Specifically, malignancies in the breast, endometrial and thyroid tissues are most common [42]. Hamartomas typically arise in epithelial tissues, such as the epidermis and mucous membranes surrounding the mouth and nose or internally in the intestinal tract [45].

Since CS presents in a myriad of different symptoms and physical manifestations, diagnosis is sometimes challenging. The International Cowden Consortium and the National Comprehensive Cancer Network (NCCN) have released diagnostic criteria for CS. According to these stipulations, CS is diagnosed if a patient presents with one or more of the following criteria [42]: 1) Pathognomonic lesions (e.g., adult Lhermitte-Duclos disease) or mucocutaneous lesions only, if there are 6 or more facial papules of which, at least 3 are tricholemmoma, or cutaneous facial papules and oral mucosal papillomatosis or oral mucosal papillomatosis and acral keratoses, or 6 or more palmoplantar keratoses; 2) Macrocephaly ($\geq 97^{th}$ percentile) in addition to another major criteria (i.e., breast carcinoma, non-medullary thyroid carcinoma, macroencephaly (megaencephaly) or endometrial carcinoma); 3) A major criterion (see list from criteria 2) and three minor criteria (i.e., non-carcinoma thyroid lesions, mental retardation (IQ $\leq$ 75), gastrointestinal hamartomas, fibrocystic disease of the breast, lipomas, fibromas, genitourinary tumors (i.e., renal cell carcinoma), genitourinary structural malformations, or uterine fibroids) or 4) Four minor criteria.

Alternatively, patients can be diagnosed with the syndrome if they present with one or more of the following [42]: 1) Pathognomonic criteria; 2) One major criteria; 3) Two minor criteria or 4) Bannayan-Riley-Ruvalcaba syndrome (BRRS).

The classic brain finding is the dysplastic cerebellar ganglicytoma (Lhermitte-Duclos disease), which is marked by a low-grade proliferation of neuronal or ganglionic cells. Only one known case of ependymoma in a patient with CS has been reported in the literature [46]. Farhadi and colleagues reported a case of a 45-year-old man who had been diagnosed with left cerebellar Lhermitte-Duclos syndrome five years prior and was suspected to have CS due to personal and familial history of hamartomas of the skin, colon polyps and lipomas. Further genetic testing confirmed that the patient had the PTEN mutation associated with CS. The patient presented with neurological symptoms of dysmetria of the left hand, headaches, spinal ataxia as well as decline in gait, and mild loss of mobility and sensation in the distal portions of both arms. Neurological examination results indicated that the patient had diminished strength and reflexes in his extremities, a negative Babinski test, dysmetria and dysdiadochokinesia on the left and notable gait ataxia. A MRI revealed the presence of a high signal intensity intramedullary ependymoma located between the C6-C7 vertebrae of the spine on a T1-weighted image. T2-weighted images revealed perifocal medullary edema, but an absence of polar cysts. Histological evaluation indicated that the mass was a WHO grade II ependymoma with epithelial, papillary and mixed cell patterns. The patient's symptoms were noted to improve over time, and nine months postoperatively, the patient's neurological symptoms had almost entirely ceased with the aid of physical therapy [41].

Von Hippel Lindau Syndrome

Von Hippel-Lindau (VHL) syndrome, an autosomal dominant condition, is marked by the development of benign and malignant neoplasms, including visceral cysts, which typically and frequently appear as retinal, spinal and cerebellar hemangioblastomas, renal cell carcinomas, pheochromocytomas, and pancreatic tumors [47]. VHL is caused by a heterozygous germline mutation in VHL tumor suppressor gene situated on chromosome 3p25-26 [48], and its prevalence is noted as 1 in 36,000 birth incidences [47]. Evidence suggests that a variation in the cyclin D1 gene (CCND1) on chromosome 11q13 may modify the phenotype [47].

Roughly 80% of those affected with VHL will develop hemangioblastomas in the brain and spinal cord, indicating that central nervous system hemangioblastomas are the prototypic lesion associated with VHL (49). Rarely, peripheral nerve hemangioblastomas may develop [50]. Manifestations of brain, spinal and retinal hemangioblastomas typically include headache, vomiting, gait disturbances, and ataxia. Spinal hemangioblastomas usually present with pain, sensory and motor loss. Seventy percent of affected individuals will present with retinal angiomas [51], while another 70% of affected individuals present with renal cell carcinoma. Approximately 5-17% of individuals develop neuroendocrine tumors [52] with 10-16% developing endolympathic sac tumors [53].

Von Hippel-Lindau phenotypes include Type 1, Type 2A, Type 2B and Type 2C [49]. VHL Type 1 is associated with retinal angiomas, CNS hemangioblastomas, renal cell carcinomas, pancreatic cysts and neuroendocrine tumors with low risk for pheochromocytomas. Hemangioblastomas, retinal angiomas and pheochromocytomas are associated with VHL Type 2 with Type 2A involving pheochromocytoma, retinal angiomas, and CNS hemangioblastomas with a low risk for renal cell carcinoma. Type 2B involves pheochromocytoma, retinal angiomas, and CNS hemangioblastomas with pancreatic cysts and neuroendocrine tumors, and include a high risk for renal carcinoma. Type 2C involves pheochromocytoma only [49].

A few cases of individuals with VHL and ependymomas have been reported, although details regarding the specifics of these cases are lacking. Neumann and Zbar briefly mentioned two patients with ependymoma in a series of 288 VHL patients [54]. Hiroshi et al. reported one ependymoma, found after molecular genetic analysis of the von Hippel-Lindau tumor suppressor gene in 38 glial tumors [48]. The remaining glial tumors consisted of six astrocytomas, one oligodendroglioma (grade II), two oligoastrocytomas, three anaplastic oligoastrocytomas (grade III), 14 anaplastic astrocytomas, and 11 glioblastoma [48]. Hiroshi et al. reported that mutations in several tumor suppressor genes were associated with the development of glial tumors.

Tuberous Sclerosis

Tuberous Sclerosis Complex (TSC) is a genetic disorder resulting from mutations within the TSC1 (coding for hamartin) and TSC2 (coding for tuberin) genes in which widespread visceral lesions potentially occur in all organ systems [55]. TSC1 and TSC2 suppress tumor development through the distinct regulation of cell growth by inhibiting the protein mammalian target of repamycin (mTOR), or FK506-binding protein 12-repamycin-associated protein 1 (FRAP1) [56]. A defect in either gene results in the lack of suppressed cell growth and ultimately lesion production. The extensive distribution of hamartin, tuberin and mTOR throughout the body provides an explanation for the array of affected organs. The estimated prevalence of TSC is 1 in 6,000 births [57].

While TSC manifests in several ways, common symptoms include early childhood or infant seizures, infantile spasms, developmental delay, skin lesions, skin abnormalities, vision problems, and kidney or lung disease. Affected individuals may present with no symptoms or may demonstrate severe symptoms including cognitive impairment, tumors and severe seizures [55]. Definite diagnosis can be made if an individual presents with two major features, or one major and two minor features. Major features include facial angiofibromas or forehead plaque, non-traumatic ungual or periungual fibroma, hypomelanotic macules (more than three), Shagreen patch (connective tissue nevus), multiple retinal nodular hamartomas, cortical tuber, subependymal nodule, subependymal giant cell astrocytoma, cardiac rhabdomyoma, single or multiple lymphangiomyomatosis lesions, and renal angiomyolipoma [58]. Minor features include multiple randomly distributed pits in dental enamel, hamartomatous rectal polyps, bone cysts, cerebral white matter migration lines, gingival fibromas, non-renal hamartoma, retinal achromic patch, "confetti" skin lesions, and multiple renal cysts. A probable diagnosis can be rendered if one major and one minor feature are present; a possible diagnosis can be made with one major symptom present or two or more minor present [58].

The most common brain manifestations of TSC include cortical tubers, the subependymal giant cell astrocytoma and subependymal hamartomas. Cortical tubers are marked by focal areas of cortical architectural disorganization (focal cortical dysplasia) often with balloon cells, gliosis and microcalcifications. Subependymal giant cell astrocytomas generally arise in the lateral ventricles and are marked by a proliferation of large astrocytic cells. The tumors are regarded as WHO grade I neoplasms. Hamartomas may be seen as small protrusions from the walls of the ventricular system. Sometimes, they are numerous and have been likened to candle guttering. They consist of disordered collections of glial cells with variable amounts of gliosis and calcification.

To our knowledge, there is only one reported case of an individual with ependymoma arising in the setting of TSC [59]; in this report, a 24-year-old white female, one week postpartum, presented with severe right-sided headaches, diplopia and blurred vision. The patient had no history of epilepsy, but had developed some cognitive impairment. Sebaceous adenomas were seen on upper cheeks and a sacral Shagreen patch was noted. The patient's left mid-finger had a periungual fibroma. Intracranial calcifications were seen in scattered areas on imaging. Radiographs of the hands demonstrated cystic areas in the distal phalanges. Ventriculography revealed tumorous protrusions into the lateral ventricles, a filling defect in the anterior horn of the right lateral ventricle with dilated lateral ventricles. The patient underwent placement of a right ventriculomastoidostomy tube. Symptoms of headache, vomiting and ataxia persisted and a craniotomy was performed with excision of a red friable tumor that filled the entire right lateral ventricle and extended to involve the foramen of Monro. A diagnosis of ependymoma was made and on the fifth postoperative day, the patient died.

REFERENCES

[1] Horn B, Heideman R, Geyer R, et al. A multi-institutional retrospective study of intracranial ependymoma in children: identification of risk factors. *J. Pediatr. Hematol. Oncol.* 1999; 21: 203-211.

[2] McLendon RE, Wiestler OD, Kros JM, et al. Ependymoma and Anaplastic Ependymoma. In WHO Classification of Tumours of the Central Nervous System. (Louis DN, Ohgaki H, Wiestler OD, et al., editors) 4th edition. IARC Press. Lyon, FR. 2007. pp. 74-80.

[3] Merchant TE, Jenkins JJ, Burger PC, et al. Influence of tumor grade on time to progression after irradiation for localized ependymoma in children. *Int. J. Radiat. Oncol. Biol. Phys*. 2002; 53: 52-57.

[4] Aguilera DG, Mazewski C, Schniederjan MJ, et al. Neurofibromatosis-2 and spinal cord ependymomas: Report of two cases and review of the literature. *Childs Nerv. Syst.* 2011; 27(5):757-764.

[5] Yokota T, Tachizawa T, Fukino K, et al. A family with spinal anaplastic ependymoma: evidence of loss of chromosome 22q in tumor. *J. Hum. Genet.* 2003; 48: 598–602.

[6] Rubio MP, Correa KM, Ramesh V, et al. Analysis of the neurofibromatosis 2 gene in human ependymomas and astrocytomas. *Cancer Res*. 1994; 54(1):45-47.

[7] Evans DG, Neurofibromatosis type 2 (NF2): A clinical and molecular review. *Orphanet J. Rare Dis*. 2009; 4:16 (doi: 10:1186/1750-1172-4-6) Accessed on September 8, 2015.

[8] Evans DG. Neurofibromatosis 2. *Gene Reviews ® 1998,* Available at http: II www.ncbi.nlm.nih.gov/books/NBK 1201/. Accessed October 8, 2015.

[9] Ruggieri M, Iannetti P, Polizzi A, et al. Earliest clinical manifestations and natural history of neurofibromatosis type 2 (NF2) in childhood: a study of 24 patients. *Neuropediatrics*. 2005; 36:21–34.

[10] Plotkin SR, O'Donnell CC, Curry Jr WT, et al. Spinal ependymomas in neurofibromatosis Type 2: a retrospective analysis of 55 patients. *J. Neurosurg. Spine*. 2011; 4: 543–547.

[11] Hagel C, Stemmer-Rachamimov AO, Bornemann A, et al. Clinical presentation, immunohistochemistry and electron microscopy indicate neurofibromatosis type 2-associated gliomas to be spinal ependymomas. *Neuropathology*. 2012; 32(6):611-616.

[12] Lim BS, Park SQ, Chang UK, et al. Spinal cord tanycytic ependymoma associated with neurofibromatosis type 2. *J. Clin. Neurosci*. 2010; 17(7):922-924.

[13] Ueki K, Sasaki T, Ishida T, et al. Spinal tanycytic ependymoma associated with Neurofibromatosis Type 2 – case report. *Neurol. Med. Chir. (Tokyo)*. 2001; 41(10):513-6.

[14] Lee M, Rezai AR, Freed D, et al. Intramedullary spinal cord tumors in Neurofibromatosis. *Neurosurgery*. 1996; 38(1):32-7.

[15] Abboud A. Neurofibromatosis type 1 (NF1). Salem Press Encyclopedia Of Health. January 2015; Available from: Research Starters, Ipswich, MA. Accessed September 21, 2015.

[16] Hongwei C, Shan M, Feng C, et al. Spinal cord ependymoma associated with Neurofibromatosis 1: Case report and review of the literature. *J. Korean Neurosurg. Soc*. 2014; 55: 43-47.

[17] Ferner RE, Huson SM, Thomas N, et al. Guidelines for the diagnosis and management of individuals with neurofibromatosis 1. *J. Med. Genet.* 2007; 44(2):81-88.
[18] Riffaud L, Vinchon M, Ragragui O, et al. Hemispheric cerebral gliomas in children with NF1: arguments for a long-term follow-up. *Childs Nerv. Syst.* 2002; 18(1), 43-47.
[19] Sharma AS, Emry ME, Metcalfe KM, et al. A case of thoracic cord ependymoma in neurofibromatosis type 1. *Endocr. Abstracts.* 2006; 12: 17.
[20] Agarwal SK, Lee Burns A, Sukhodolets KE, et al. Molecular pathology of the MEN1 gene. *Ann. N.Y. Acad. Sci.* 2004; 1014: 189-198.
[21] Thakker RV. Multiple endocrine neoplasia type 1. *Endocrinol. Metab. Clin. North Am.* 2000; 29: 541-567.
[22] Giusti F, Marini F, Brandi ML. Multiple endocrine neoplasia type I. GeneReviews [Internet] (Pagon RA, Adam MP, Ardinger HH, et al., editors). Seattle, WA. http://www.ncbi.nlm.nih.gov/books/NBK1538/. Accessed June 24, 2015.
[23] Asgharian B, Chen Y-J, Patronas NJ, et al. Meningiomas may be a component tumor of multiple endocrine neoplasia type I. *Clin. Cancer Res.* 2004; 10: 869-880.
[24] Kato H, Uchimura I, Morohoshi M, et al. Multiple endocrine neoplasia type I associated with spinal ependymoma. *Int. Med.* 1996; 35(4): 285-289.
[25] Giraud S, Choplin H, Teh BT, et al. A large multiple endocrine neoplasia type I family with clinical expression suggestive of anticipation. *J. Clin. Endocrinol. Metab.*1997; 82 (10): 3487-3492.
[26] Al-Salameh A, Francois P, Giraud S, et al. Intracranial ependymoma associated with multiple endocrine type 1. *J. Endocrinol. Invest.* 2010; 33(5): 353-356.
[27] Funayama T, Sakane M, Yoshizawa T, et al. Tanycytic ependymoma of the filum terminale associated with multiple endocrine neoplasia type I: first reported case. *Spine J.* 2013; 13: e49-e54.
[28] Spaulding R, Alatassi H, Metzinger DS, et al. Ependymoma and carcinoid tumor associated with ovarian mature cystic teratoma in a patient with multiple endocrine neoplasia I. *Case Rep. Obstet. Gynecol.*2014; Article ID 712657. Accessed August 5, 2015.
[29] Sarin S, Bernath A. Turcot syndrome (glioma polyposis): a case report. South Med. J. 2008; 101(12):1273-1274.
[30] Turcot Syndrome. *Cancer. Net.* Available at: http://www.cancer.net/cancer-types/turcot-syndrome. Accessed August 10, 2015.
[31] Hamilton SR, Liu B, Parsons RE, Papadopoulos N, Jen J, Powell SM et al. The molecular basis of Turcot's syndrome. *New Engl. J. Med.* 1995; 332(13): 839-847.
[32] Torres CF, Korones DN, Pilcher W. Multiple ependymomas in a patient with Turcot's syndrome. *Med. Pediatr. Oncol.* 1997; 28(1):59-61.
[33] Mullins KJ, Rubio A, Myers SP, et al. Malignant ependymomas in a patient with Turcot's syndrome: case report and management guidelines. Surg. Neurol. 1998; 49(8):290-294.
[34] Rieber J, Remke M, Hartmann C, et al. Novel oncogene amplifications in tumors from a family with Li-Fraumeni syndrome. Genes Chromo. Canc. 2009; 48(7):558-568.
[35] Pantziarka, P. Primed for cancer: Li Fraumeni syndrome and the pre-cancerous niche. Ecancermedicalscience 2015; 9: 541. Accessed August 15, 2015.
[36] Li-Fraumeni syndrome. *Genetics Home Reference* 2015. Available at: http://ghr.nlm.nih.gov/condition/li-fraumeni-syndrome/show/print. Accessed August 15, 2015.

[37] Ilić MP, Kiralj A, Markov B, et al. Li-Fraumeni syndrome: A case report. Vojnosanit Pregl 2014; 71(12):1159-1162.

[38] Li-Fraumeni Syndrome. *Cancer. Net.* 2012. Available at: http://www.cancer.net/cancer-types/li-fraumeni-syndrome. Accessed August 15, 2015.

[39] Lloyd II KM, Dennis M. Cowden's disease: a possible new symptom complex with multiple system involvement. *Ann. Intern. Med.* 1963; 58(1):136-142.

[40] Nelen MR, Kremer H, Konings IBM, et al. Novel PTEN mutations in patients with Cowden disease: absence of clear genotype-phenotype correlations. *Eur. J. Hum. Genet.* 1999; 7(3):267-273.

[41] Gustafson S, Zbuk KM, Scacheri C, et al. Cowden syndrome. *Semin. Oncol.* 2007; 34(5):428-434.

[42] Farooq A, Walker LJ, Bowling J, et al. Cowden syndrome. *Cancer Treat. Rev.* 2010; 36(8):577-583.

[43] Nelen MR, Padberg GW, Peters EA, et al. Localization of the gene for Cowden disease to chromosome10q22-23. *Nat. Genet.* 1996; 13(1): 114-116.

[44] Li DM, Sun H. TEP1, encoded by a candidate tumor suppressor locus, is a novel protein tyrosine phosphatase regulated by transforming growth factor ß. *Cancer Res.* 1997;57(11):2124-2129.

[45] Cowden syndrome. *Genetics Home Reference* 2015. Available at: http://ghr.nlm.nih.gov/condition/cowden-syndrome. Accessed August 15, 2015.

[46] Farhadi MR, Rittierodt M, Stan A, et al. Intramedullary ependymoma associated with Lhermitte-Duclos disease and Cowden syndrome. *Clin. Neurol. Neurosurg.* 2007; 109(8): 692-697.

[47] Online Mendelian Inheritance in Man, OMIM®. McKusick-Nathans Institute of Genetic Medicine, Johns Hopkins University (Baltimore, MD), World Wide Web URL: http://omim.org/. Accessed August 1, 2015.

[48] Kanno H, Shuin T, Kondo K, et al. Somatic mutations of the von Hippel-Lindau tumor suppressor gene and loss of heterozygosity on chromosome 3p in human glial tumors. *Cancer Res.* 1997; 57, 1035-1038.

[49] Frantzen C, Klasson TD, Links TP, et al. Von Hippel-Lindau Syndrome. 2000 May 17 In: Pagon RA, Adam MP, Ardinger HH, et al., editors. *Gene Reviews*. Seattle (WA): University of Washington, Seattle; 1993-2015.

[50] Giannini C, Scheithauer BW, Hellbusch LC, et al. Peripheral nerve hemangioblastoma. *Mod. Pathol.* 1998;11(10):999–1004.

[51] Webster AR, Maher ER, Moore AT. Clinical characteristics of ocular angiomatosis in von Hippel-Lindau disease and correlation with germline mutation. *Arch. Ophthalmol.* 1999; 117(3):371–378.

[52] Lonser RR, Butman JA, Huntoon K, et al. Prospective natural history study of central nervous system hemangioblastomas in von Hippel-Lindau disease. *J. Neurosurg.* 2014; 120(5):1055–1062.

[53] Kim HJ, Butman JA, Brewer C, et al. Tumors of the endolymphatic sac in patients with von Hippel- Lindau disease: implications for their natural history, diagnosis, and treatment. *J. Neurosurg.* 2005; 102(3):503–512.

[54] Neumann HP, Zbar B. Renal cysts, renal cancer and von Hippel-Lindau disease. *Kidney Int.* 1997; 51(1): 16-26.

[55] Mavris M. Tuberous Sclerosis. Salem Press Encyclopedia Of Health. January 2014; Available from: Research Starters, Ipswich, MA. Accessed July 14, 2015.

[56] Cabrera-López C, Bullich G, Marti TO, et al. Insight into response to mTOR inhibition when PKD1 and TSC2 are mutated. BMC Medical Genetics [serial online]. June 17, 2015;16:39. Available from: MEDLINE with Full Text, Ipswich, MA. Accessed July 22, 2015.

[57] About TSC. Tuberous Sclerosis Alliance website. Available at http://www.tsalliance.org. Accessed July 13, 2015.

[58] Northup H, Krueger D. The international Tuberous Sclerosis Complex Consensus Group. Tuberous sclerosis complex diagnostic criteria update: Recommendations of the 2012 International Tuberous Sclerosis Complex Consensus Conference. *Pediatr. Neurol.* 2013; 49(4); 243-254.

[59] MacCarty WJ, Russel DG. Tuberous sclerosis: report of a case with ependymoma. *Radiology*. 1958; 71(6): 833-839.

In: Ependymomas
Editor: Raquel Fowler

ISBN: 978-1-63484-405-5

Chapter 6

EPENDYMOMA IN CHILDREN: CURRENT TREATMENT STRATEGIES AND EVOLVING MOLECULAR BIOLOGY

Soumen Khatua**, MD
Pediatric Neuro-Oncology, Pediatric Brain Tumor Program,
Children's Cancer Hospital, The University of Texas,
MD Anderson Cancer Center, Houston, TX, US

ABSTRACT

Ependymomas are the third commonest tumor of the central nervous system (CNS) accounting for 6-12% of brain tumors in children. Even with advances in neurosurgical, neuroimaging and postoperative adjuvant therapy, the prognosis remains poor with a 5 year progression free survival (PFS) of 23-45%. Recurrence of tumor develops in 50% of cases, even after complete surgical resection followed by radiotherapy. To-date no chemotherapeutic regimen has proven to be of significant clinical benefit. Predicting tumor behavior and defining robust correlates of disease outcome based on histopathology and clinical characteristics remains suboptimal. Paucity of cell lines, failure to develop animal models of these tumors unlike other CNS malignancies, has precluded better understanding of the oncogenic drivers, undermining development of targeted therapy. Thus these tumors have remained therapeutically frustrating and enigmatic. However, over the last few years major breakthrough in the understanding of the molecular biology and subtypes, cellular origin of these tumor cells and signaling pathways are now providing insights into development of biological targeted therapies in ependymoma. It is now clear that even with histopathological similarities, these are genetically heterogeneous tumors with diverse clinical outcomes. Rapid evolution of data now suggests three principal molecular subgroups of ependymomas in children, based on gene clustering. These include supratentorial (ST), posterior fossa (PF) and the spinal (SP) and posterior fossa (PF) subtypes. More recently based on transcriptome profiling, two subgroups (Group A and B) of PF ependymomas have been identified with distinct molecular, clinical characteristics and specific chromosomal aberrations. Signaling pathways specific to these subtypes have now been delineated, raising hopes of defining therapeutic targets. In the years ahead sustained research endeavors are needed to

* 713.792.3280 (P). 713.792.0608 (F). Email: skhatua@mdanderson.org.

enhance our understanding of the elusive biology of these tumors. This will enable us to profile optimal biologically driven targeted therapy in addition to conventional treatment modalities to improve survival rate.

INTRODUCTION

Ependymomas are the third most common pediatric tumor of the central nervous system (CNS), accounting for 6-12% of brain tumors in children [1]. These tumors can occur anywhere in the neuraxis and arise from the ependymal lining of the ventricles and the central canal. In children nearly 90% of these malignancies are intracranial of which two-thirds arise from the posterior fossa (infratentorial) and one-third is located in the supratentorial area [2, 3]. Currently these tumors are classified into three grades by the World Health Organization; (WHO) grade I (subependymomas and myxopapillary), Grade II (classic) and Grade III asanaplastic type [4]. This classification has remained controversial due to the inherent subjectivity, mostly between the classic and anaplastic variants noted with inter-observer variability. Also prognostic outcomes based on histological grading, has remained diverse in different clinical trials, undermining the current histopathological grading to a certain extent [5]. Current management of these tumors has remained the same over the last two decades, with surgery followed by radiation therapy as an adjuvant strategy. The role of chemotherapy has remained uncertain and controversial. Considered as a surgical disease, complete resection has been the most favorable consistent prognostic factor [6]. However recurrences can develop in 50% of the tumors after gross total resection and adjuvant radiotherapy [7, 8]. Even with advancements in the multidisciplinary management of brain tumors prognosis remains poor in these malignancies. The 5 year progression free survival (PFS) and overall survival (OS) is 23-45% and 50-70% respectively, and late relapses known to occur even after a decade makes these tumors therapeutically formidable [9, 10]. The elusive biology of these tumors had prevented development of clinical trials geared towards targeted therapy, resulting in clinical failures. Recent revelations are providing novel insights into the genomic/epigenomic biology of these tumors, which now temper enthusiasm to profile newer therapeutics. This chapter will discuss the current management of pediatric ependymomas and the evolving biological data.

EPIDEMIOLOGY

More than half of these tumors occur in younger children less than 5 years and are prevalent twice as common in males [11]. Unlike adults where most of these tumors occur in the spine, children have age-specific locations. Infratentorial tumors tend to occur in younger children while spinal and supratentorial ependymoma predominate in the older age group [12]. The etiology of ependymomas remains obscure with no robust correlations between environmental or infectious etiology. Few non-specific data shows the SV40 virus is capable of inducing brain tumors including ependymomas [13]. Neurofibromatosis type 2 (NF2) is the only known genetic defect with a predisposition to develop these tumors, with nearly 25-70% of sporadic intraspinal ependymomas harboring NF2 mutations [14].

HISTOPATHOLOGICAL CHARACTERISTICS

Ependymomas are classified into three grades and four histological variants (Table 1). The most common histopathological subtypes occurring in children are classic ependymoma (Grade II) and anaplastic ependymoma (Grade III). The distinction between the two grades is difficult and lack reproducibility, with discordance between neuropathologists being as high as 69% [15]. Anaplastic variants have higher cellularity, nuclear atypia, frequent mitosis and variable degrees of vascular proliferation and necrosis. Classic ependymomas exhibit perivascular pseudorosettes, and are less cellular with minimal mitotic activity and may demonstrate nuclear atypia. Three subtypes are noted in this grade which includes cellular, papillary and the clear-cell variants. Grade I include two subtypes: myxopapillary ependymoma (MPE) and subependymoma, both of which are rare in children. MPE are slow growing tumors and occur almost exclusively in the caudaequina, originating from the filumterminale, with a predisposition to spread in other parts of the CNS in children. Subependymoma is a rarer variant of Grade I ependymoma seen in <1% of children, and have a low proliferation index (MIB-1). They have an excellent prognosis following surgical resection [16, 17].

TREATMENT

Therapeutic strategy for pediatric ependymomas includes maximal safe surgical resection, followed by adjuvant therapy. This includes in most cases radiation with or without chemotherapy.

SURGERY

Local control is most important to prevent recurrence as these tumors are locally invasive with low metastatic potential and leptomeningeal dissemination seen only in 7-12% of cases at diagnosis. Thus a safe gross total resection (GTR) is aimed with intent to remove macroscopical disease [18]. This could be challenging in eloquent areas of the brain including posterior fossa tumors, and yet be able to preserve neurovascular integrity. Thus GTR has been achievable in only 40-66% of cases, mostly in supratentorial tumors in contrast to posterior fossa ependymomas [19, 20]. Historically though GTR is consistently reported as the most favorable prognostic factor, some studies have refuted this and recurrences have been seen in up to 50% cases, mostly in posterior fossa tumors even after GTR and adjuvant radiotherapy [21, 22].

RADIATION THERAPY

Though no randomized trial has been performed comparing radiation therapy following surgery versus surgery alone in pediatric ependymomas, historically patients who have received radiation therapy to the tumor bed with a dose of 54 to 59.4 Gy as an adjuvant treatment have fared better [23]. A study in 22 children who received intensity modulated radiotherapy (IMRT) following surgical resection, showed a 3 year EFS and OS of 68 and 87% respectively [24]. Another study of 78 children less than 3 years treated with adjuvant 3D- conformal radiotherapy (CRT) after surgical resection had a 7 year EFS and OS of 69.1 and 81% respectively [25]. These outcomes reflect improved survival in comparison to historical controls. The emerging role and benefits of proton beam radiation in pediatric CNS tumors are beginning to surface; its evaluation in pediatric ependymomas needs to be further explored [26]. Currently the Children's Oncology Group (COG) ACNS 0831 is evaluating the outcome of adjuvant radiotherapy in all children with anaplastic histology irrespective of location, and in all posterior fossa ependymomas. This study is also evaluating the outcome of "observation only" strategy in patients with supratentorial non-anaplastic ependymomas who have undergone a GTR of the tumor. This is based on good outcomes seen with a low 5 year mortality following surgery, without any adjuvant radiotherapy in smaller studies [27, 28]. Hyper fractionated radiotherapy has been proposed and evaluated in some studies, but to date no objective evidence of benefit has been seen with increased dose of radiation [29]. The role of craniospinal irradiation is reserved for patients with neuraxis dissemination, but no long term evaluation of benefits and survival has been robustly concluded [30].

Chemotherapy

Chemotherapy has been evaluated in pediatric ependymoma, but itrole remains controversial though benefits have been noted in a subset of patients. In the CCG942 randomized study, children received PCV (procarbazine, CCNU, vincristine) regimen following radiation therapy, versus no adjuvant chemotherapy after irradiation. No benefits were noted with addition of chemotherapy [31]. In the CCG921 two arms of chemotherapy were used (PCV versus 8-in-1 which included vincristine, hydroxurea, procarbazine, CCNU, cisplatin, cytarabine and methylprednisolone), with neither regimen showing improved survival benefit [32]. Subsequent studies by the United Kingdom Cancer and Leukemia Group (UKCCSG) and the International Society of Pediatric Oncology (SIOP) evaluated the outcome of postoperative chemotherapy in children with ependymoma. In younger children who did not receive radiation therapy, a 5 year OS of 63.4% was noted in patients without metastatic disease, suggesting a likely role of chemotherapy [33]. The current COG trial ACNS0821 (NCT01096368) is prospectively evaluating the role of chemotherapy regimen with vincristine, cisplatin, etoposide and cyclophosphamide following subtotal resection of tumors, and the feasibility of a second-look surgery after chemotherapy, and also evaluating the role of post-radiation maintenance chemotherapy with an observation arm after radiation. This is based on data of a subset of children with these tumors showing benefit with chemotherapy. In the CCG 9942 study, 57% of patients treated with chemotherapy showed variable tumor responses (40% had complete response and 17% partial response) allowing second-look surgery [34]. The Head Start III trial demonstrated a 3 year PFS of 86% in supratentorial tumors treated versus 27% in infratentorial tumors using a myeloablative chemotherapeutic regimen [35].

The evolving genomic/epigenomic data in pediatric ependymoma, as described in the next section, shows significant heterogeneity of the molecular biology, based on age and location of tumors. This now throws light on the reason for diverseness of clinical response, unpredictable relapses noted in these trials.

GENETIC LANDSCAPE OF EPENDYMOMA

Over the last few years a surge in the revelation of putative immunohistochemical and genomic markers have surfaced, which is beginning to throw light on the biology of these tumors, reasons for diverse clinical outcome and clues to novel therapeutics. Before the advent of genomic era, karytopic analysis revealed the range of complex profile of structural and numerical aberration of pediatric ependymomas. Chromosomal alterations occur in 60% of pediatric ependymomas, much less frequently than seen in adults. Most frequent chromosomal aberrations seen in pediatric ependymomas are gain of chromosome 1q, 7 and 9 and loss of chromosome 22, 3, 9p, 13q, 6q, 1p, 17 and 6. Gain of 1q and loss of chromosome 22 is common in recurrent ependymoma and suggest that these aberrations are a potential marker of aggressive disease [36, 37]. The biological heterogeneity of these tumors is further reaffirmed by location-specific differences. Pediatric spinal ependymoma demonstrate whole chromosomal imbalances which include gains of chromosome of 7, 9, 11, 18 and 20 or loss of chromosome 1, 2 and 10. This is in contrast to intracranial ependymomas which show gain of chromosome of 1q, and loss of chromosome 22, 3, 9p and 13q [38, 39]. The advent of array comparative genomic hybridization (aCGH) has enabled more subtle identification of genomic aberrations. Children average 3.8 genomic abnormalities per tumor, as opposed to 7.5 in adults [40]. A balanced genomic profile without any chromosomal gain or loss is prevalent in 36-58% of pediatric ependymomas, seen more commonly in younger children. A compendium of CGH and DNA cytometry studies has shown associations between lower histological grade and favorable outcome in patient with higher number of genomic anomalies. This likely explains the worse prognosis in younger children (<3 years) who have a more balanced or a silent genomic structure [41, 42].

Immunohistocehmical methodology has identified some important prognostic markers in these tumors. Increased expression of p53, bcl-2 and cyclin D labeling index of >5%, is associated with a worse PFS (43-45). High Ki-67/MIB1 labeling index is associated with a poor OS and increased tendency of tumor dissemination to the cerebrospinal fluid (CSF) (46). Immunohistochemical assay of 59 ependymal tumors revealed that ERBB2/ERBB4 co-expression with raised Ki-67, was associated with poor survival outcome. However ERBB2/ERBB4 co-expression alone did not correlate with poor outcome [47].

Telemorase maintenance and its lengthening which is known to sustain oncogenesis are seen in many malignancies, including pediatric tumors. It is now known that it functions as a homodimer, containing a catalytic component with reverse transcriptase activity (hTERT). Expression of hTERT and its nuclear chaperone nucleolin are important prognostic markers in childhood ependymoma [48]. The gene encoding hTERT located on chromosome 5p13.3 is amplified in intracranial ependymomas suggesting this interlinked group could be a strong driver of tumor formation [49]. The tenascin c (TNC) gene on chromosome 9is upregulated in infant ependymomas, and its intracellular accumulation is identified as a poor prognostic marker in these tumors [50].

Genomic analysis of ependymoma showed a gain of 1q (1q21-32) being associated with a worse OS and increased tendency for recurrence. This accumulation is more common in posterior fossa tumors with anaplastic histology [51]. Recurrent gain at 1q23.3 which contains the gene *DUSP1* is known to play a role in cell proliferation and a potential oncogene. Further dissection of locus 1q21-32 identified genes of further interest including *CHI3L1*, whose amplification correlates with tumor recurrence and its protein expression with tumor necrosis [52, 53]. Smaller studies have elucidated the prognostic role of genes such as *NRXN2, TPR, SEMA5, NRCAM, CDK4 and ADRM1*, though larger prospective studies are needed to validate these findings [54]. Study using gene expression profiling identified, 3-gene subset *PLEK* (pleckstrin), *NF-kappaB2* (nuclear factor kappa beta-2), and *LOC374491* (TPTE and PTEN homologous inositol phosphatase pseudogene), which could be predictor of tumor recurrence [55]. Pediatric posterior fossa ependymomas also overexpress c-myc, implicating Notch pathway activation in tumorogenesis and making *NOTCH1* and *NOTCH4* targetable putative oncogenes [56]. Upregulation of several components of the EPHB-EPHRIN and NOTCH signaling as well as deletion of *Ink4a/ARF* are noted in subsets of supratentorial ependymoma [57]. High expression of *HOXB5*, *PLA2G5*, and *ITIH2* have been shown to distinguish grade I spinal ependymomas from intracranial tumors and the expression of these genes known to be involved in apoptosis, angiogenesis, signal transduction and tumor invasiveness can be potentially used to distinguish grade I from grade II and grade III intracranial ependymomas. However these initial findings were not consistently reproducible and did not reaffirm the differences in molecular expression, between tumors located in the posterior fossa and in other sites [58].

Recent landmark findings in pediatric ependymoma using large collaborative genome-scale efforts have identified reproducible evidence of distinct molecular subtypes of ependymomas. Using DNA methylation profiling, subgroups have been discerned in three locations (supratentorial (ST), posterior fossa (PF) and spinal cord (SP)). This has now provided some novel biological insights into the intriguing nature of these malignancies.

Two molecular different subtypes within the posterior fossa which are histologically similar are now clearly defined. These types differ based on the age, transcriptional, genomic, epigenetic profile and clinical outcome [59]. These include Group A, labelled as *PF-EPN-A* and Group B known as *PF-EPN-B*.

PF-EPN-A subtypes are seen in younger children and infants (median age of 2.5 years), show a quieter genome with no recurrent gene alterations. However epigenetic analysis identified increased DNA methylation of aunique gene involved in cell differentiation, commonly termed as CpG island methylator phenotype (CIMP). Epigenetic silencing of CIMP, are same as those silenced by the Polycomb repressive complex 2 (PRC2) in embryonic stem cells. This phenomenon is believed to result in maintaining Gr A tumors in a primitive stage and ensuing ongoing oncogenesis [60, 61]. H3K27 trimethylation known to down-regulate differentiation genes are notably present in tumors in this region. Also noted are activation of critical oncogenic signaling pathways (vascular endothelial growth factor (VEGF), platelet derived growth factor receptor (PDGFR), integrin and the MAPK in this subtype [62]. These results temper enthusiasm in profiling treatment strategies that target DNA CpG methylation, PRC2 and histone deacetylase. Though known to be gnomically relatively stable, nearly 25% of these tumors show gain of chromosome 1q, known to be a negative prognostic factor, correlating the known relatively poor outcome of posterior fossa tumors [63]. These oncogenes and activation of various pathways render poor prognosis for Gr A tumors with increased tendency to recur. Role of Interleukin-6/STAT3 pathway driving an inflammatory phenotype in these Gr A tumors is now postulated, raising the possibility of this pathway being a therapeutic target [64].

PF-EPN-B occurs in older children and young adults, and has an improved outcome. In contrast to the Gr A tumors they display significant genomic aberrations. They demonstrate increased copy number variations including gains of 9q, 15q and 18q and loss of 6q and 22q. These chromosomal aberrations are associated with better prognosis and a 5 year PFS and OS of 73% and 100% respectively [40, 59].

Supratentorial Ependymoma

Two subtypes of tumors in this location, originating by tumorigenic gene fusions are *ST-EPN-RELA* and *ST-EPN-YAP1* are now known to occur with well-defined molecular differences.

ST-EPN-RELA occurs in younger children and exhibit significant chromosome aberrations. Gene fusion between the *C11 orf95* and *RELA* was noted in nearly 70% of tumors in this location. This resulted in up-regulation of the NF-kB signaling known to drive tumorogenesis. These children have a poor clinical outcome [65].

ST-EPN-YAP1 is less common, occurring in very young children and has a favorable survival outcome. The YAP1 fusion protein also known to drive NOTCH signaling holds promise as a druggable target and needs further evaluation [59].

Spinal Ependymoma (SP)

These are very rare in children and are subtyped as SP-subependymoma, SP-myxopapillary and SP-EPN. These usually have a balanced genome and carry a good prognosis.

Conclusion

Pediatric ependymoma has remained a *surgical tumor* with a poor prognosis. This is due to its elusive biology, increased rate of recurrence and lack of targeted therapy. The changing paradigm of research focus and ameliorated understanding of the heterogeneous genomic landscape of ependymomas, are now providing novel treatment insights. The future tasks and challenge lies ahead in effectively translating this fast-paced evolving biology, into the most effective targeted therapy in compendium with conventional treatment strategies, as we look forward to a new era in the management of these formidable tumors.

REFERENCES

[1] Ostrom Q. T., de Blank P. M., Kruchko C. et al. (2015). Alex Lemonade Stand Foundation Infant and Childhood Primary Brain and Central Nervous System Tumors Diagnosed in the United States in 2007-2011. *Neuro Oncol.* 16 Suppl 10: x1-x36. doi:10.1093/neuonc/nou327.

[2] Wiestler O. D., Schiffer D., Coons S. W., Prayson R. A., Rosenblum M. K. *Ependymoma: Pathology and genetics of tumors of the central nervous system.* Lyon: IARC; 2000.

[3] Merchant T. E, Fouladi M. (2005). New therapeutic approaches including radiation and chemotherapy. *J Neurooncol.* 75(3):287-99.

[4] Louis D. N., Ohgaki H., Wiestler O. D. et al. (2007). The 2007 WHO classification of tumors of the central nervous system. *Acta Neuropathol.* 114(2):97-109.

[5] Merchant T. E., Jenkins J. J., Burger P. C. et al. (2002). Influence of tumor grade on time to progression after irradiation for localized ependymoma in children. *Int J Radiat Oncol Biol Phys.* 53(1):52-7.

[6] Horn B., Heideman R., Geyer R. et al. (1999). A multi-institutional retrospective study of intracranial ependymoma in children: identification of risk factors. *J Pediatr Hematol Oncol.* 21(3): 203-211.

[7] Antony R., Wong K. E., Patel M. et al. (2014). A retrospective analysis of recurrent intracranial ependymoma. *Pediatr Blood Cancer.* 61(7): 1195-1201. doi:10.1002/pbc.24996.

[8] Kawabata Y., Takahashi J. A., Arakawa Y. et al. (2005). Long-term outcome in patients harboring intracranial ependymoma. *J Neurosurg.* 103(1):31-37.

[9] Zacharoulis S., Levy A., Chi S. N. et al. (2007). Outcome for young children newly diagnosed with ependymoma, treated with intensive induction chemotherapy followed by myeloablative chemotherapy and autologous stem cell rescue. *Pediatr Blood Cancer.* 49(1):34-40.

[10] Cage T. A., Clark A. J., Aranda D. et al. (2013). A systematic review of treatment outcomes in pediatric patients with intracranial ependymomas. *J Neurosurg Pediatr.* 11(6):673-81. doi:10.3171/2013.2.PEDS12345.

[11] Rodríguez D., Cheung M. C., Housri N. et al. (2009). Outcome of malignant CNS ependymomas: an examination of 2408 cases through the Surveillance, *Epidemiology, and End Results* (SEER) database (1973-2005). 156(2):340-51. doi:10.1016/j.jss.2009.04.024.

[12] McGuire C. S., Sainani K. L., Fisher P. G. et al. Incidence patterns for ependymoma: a surveillance, epidemiology, and end results study. *J Neurosurg.* 110(4):725-729. doi:10.3171/2008.9.JNS08117.

[13] Reuther F. J., Löhler J., Herms J. et al. (2001). Low incidence of SV40-like sequences in ependymal tumors. *J Pathol.* 195(5):580-585.

[14] Plotkin S. R., O'Donnell C. C., Curry W. T. et al. (2011). Spinal ependymomas in neurofibromatosis Type 2: a retrospective analysis of 55 patients. *J Neurosurg Spine.* 14(4):543-7. doi:10.3171/2010.11. SPINE103 50.

[15] Ellison D. W., Kocak M., Figarella-Branger D. et al. (2011). Histopathological grading of pediatric ependymoma: reproducibility and clinical relevance in European trial cohorts. *J Neqat Results Biomed.* 10:7. doi:10.1186/1477-5751-10-7.

[16] McLendon R. E., Wiestler O. D., Kros J. M. et al. *Ependymoma.* In: Louis D. N., Ohgaki H., Wiestler O. D., Cavanee W. K. eds. Pathology and Genetics of Tumors of the Nervous System. 3rd ed. Lyon: IARC; 2007:72-80.

[17] Rushing E. J., Cooper P. B., Quezado M. (2007) et al. Subependymoma revisited: c; inicopathological evaluation of 83 cases. *J Neurooncol.* 85(3): 297-305.

[18] McLaughlin M. P., Marcus R. B. Jr., Buatti J. M. et al. (1998). Ependymoma: results, prognostic factors and treatment recommendations. *Int J* Radiat *Oncol Biol Phys* 40(4):845-850.

[19] Pollack I. F., Gerszten P. C., Martinez A. J. et al. (1995). Intracranial ependymomas of childhood: long-term outcome and prognostic factors. *Neurosurgery.* 37(4):655-66. Discussion 666-667.

[20] Duffner P. K., Krischer J. P., Sanford R. A. et al. (1998). Prognostic factors in infants and very young children with intracranial ependymomas. *Pediatr Neurosurg* 28(4):215-22.

[21] Goldwein J. W., Leahy J. M., Packer R. J. et al. (1990). Intracranial ependymomas in children. *Int J Radiat Oncol Biol Phys* 19:1497-502.

[22] Sowar K., Straessle J., Donson A. M. et al. (2006). Predicting which children are at risk for ependymoma relapse. *J Neurooncol* 78:41-46.

[23] Swanson E. L., Amdur R. J., Morris C. G. et al. (2011). Intracranial ependymomas treated with radiotherapy: long term results from a single institution. *J Neurooncol.* 102(3):451-457. doi:10.1007/s11060-010-0344-0.

[24] Schroeder T. M., Chintagumpala M., Okcu M. F. (2008). Intensity-modulated radiation therapy in childhood ependymoma. *Int J Radiat Oncol Biol Phys* 71(4):987-93. doi: 10.1016/j.ijrobp.2007.11.058.

[25] Merchant T. E., Li C., Xiong X. (2009). Conformal radiotherapy after surgery for pediatric ependymoma: a prospective study. *Lancet Oncol* 10(3):258-66.

[26] MacDonald S. M., Safai S., Trofimov A. et al. (2008). Proton radiotherapy for childhood ependymoma: initial clinical outcomes and dose comparisons. *Int J Radiat Oncol Biol Phys* 71(4):979-86. doi:10. 1016/j.ijrobp.2007.

[27] Hukin J., Epstein F., Lefton D., Allen J. (1998). Treatment of intracranial ependymoma by surgery alone. *Pediatr Neurosurg* 29(1): 40-45.

[28] Aizer A. A., Ancukiewicz M., Nguyen P. L. et al. (2013). Natural history and role of radiation in patients with supratentorial and infratentorial WHO Grade II ependymomas: results from a population based study. *J Neurooncol* 115(3):411-9. doi:10.1007/s11060-013-1237-1239.

[29] Conter C., Carrie C., Bernier V. (2009). Intracranial ependymomas in children: society of pediatric oncology experience with postoperative hyper fractionated local radiotherapy. *Int J Radiat Oncol Biol Phys.* 74(5): 1536-1542. doi: 10.1016/j.ijrobp.2008.09.051.

[30] Zacharoulis S., Ji L., Pollack I. F. et al. (2008). Metastatic ependymoma: a multi-institutional retrospective analysis of prognostic factors. *Pediatr Blood Cancer.* 50(2):231-235.

[31] Evans A. E., Anderson J. R., Lefkowitz-Boudreaux I. B. et al. (1996). Adjuvant chemotherapy of childhood posterior fossa ependymoma: cranio-spinal irradiation with or without adjuvant CCNU, vincristine, and prednisone: a Children's Cancer Group study. *Med Pediatr Oncol*. 27(1):8-14.
[32] Robertson P. L., Zeltzer P. M., Boyett J. M. et al. (1998). Survival and prognostic factors following radiation therapy and chemotherapy for ependymomas in children: a report of the Children's Cancer Group. *J Neurosurg*. 88(4):695-703.
[33] Grundy R. G., Wilne S. A., Weston C. L. et al. (2007). Primary postoperative chemotherapy without radiotherapy for intracranial ependymoma in children: the UKCCSG/SIOP prospective study. *Lancet Oncol*. 8(8):696-705.
[34] Garvin J. H. Jr., Selch M. T., Holmes E. et al. (2012). Phase II study of pre-irradiation chemotherapy for childhood intracranial ependymoma. Children's Cancer Group protocol 9942: a report from the Children's Oncology Group. *Pediatr Blood Cancer*. 2012 59(7):1183-1189. doi:10. 1002/pbc.24274.
[35] Venkatramani R., Ji L., Lasky J. (2013). Outcome of infants and young children with newly diagnosed ependymoma treated on the "Head Start" III prospective clinical trial. *J Neurooncol*. 113(2):285-291.doi:10.1007/s 11060-013-1111-9.
[36] Kilday J. P., Rahman R., Dyer S. et al. (2009). Pediatric ependymoma: biological perspectives. *Mol Cancer Res*. 7(6):765-86. doi:10.1158/1541-7786.MCR-08-0584.
[37] Carter M., Nicholson J., Ross F. et al. 2002. Genetic abnormalities detected in ependymomas by comparative genomic hybridisation. *Br J Cancer*. 86(6): 929-939.
[38] Pezzolo A., Capra V., Raso A. et al. (2008). *Identification of novel chromosomal abnormalities and prognostic cytogenetics markers in intracranial pediatric ependymoma*. 261(2):235-243. doi:10.1016/j. canlet.2007.11.021.
[39] Shlomit R., Ayala A. G., Michal D. et al. (2000). *Gains and losses of DNA sequences in childhood brain tumors analyzed by comparative genomic hybridization*. 121(1):67-72.
[40] Modena P., Lualdi E., Facchinetti F. et al. (2006). *Identification of tumor-specific molecular signatures in intracranial ependymoma and association with clinical characteristics*. 24(33):5223-5233.
[41] Gilhuis H. J., van der Laak J., Wesseling P. et al. (2004). Inverse correlation between genetic aberrations and malignancy grade in ependymal tumors: a paradox? *J Neurooncol*. 66(1-2):111-116.
[42] Dyer S., Prebble E., Davison V. et al. (2002). Genomic imbalances in pediatric intracranial ependymomas define clinically relevant groups. *Am J Pathol*. 161(6):2133-2141.
[43] Zamecnik J., Snuderl M., Eckschlager T. et al. (2003). Pediatric intracranial ependymomas: prognostic relevance of histological, immunohistochemical, and flow cytometric factors. *Mod Pathol*. 16(10): 980-991.
[44] Verstegen M. J., Leenstra D. T., Ijlst-Keizers H. et al. (2002). Proliferation and apoptosis-related proteins in intracranial ependymomas: an immunohistochemical analysis. *J Neurooncol*. 56:21-28.
[45] Rushing E. J., Brown D. F., Hladik C. L. et al. (1998). Correlation of bcl-2, p53 and MIB-1 expression with ependymoma grade and subtype. *Mod Pathol*. 11(5):464-470.
[46] Suzuki S., Oka H., Kawano N. et al. (2001). Prognostic value of Ki-67 (MIB-1) and p53 in ependymomas. *Brain Tumor Pathol*. 18(2):151-4.

[47] Gilbertson R. J., Bentley L., Hernan R. et al. (2002). ERBB receptor signaling promotes ependymoma cell proliferation and represents a potential novel therapeutic target for this disease. *Clin Cancer Res.* 8(10):3054-3064.

[48] Ridley L., Rahman R., Brundler M. A. et al. (2008). Multifactorial analysis of predictors of outcome in pediatric intracranial ependymoma. *Neuro Oncol.* 10(5):675-689. doi:10.1215/15228517-2008-036.

[49] Mendrzyk F., Korshunov A., Benner A. et al. (2006). Identification of gains of 1q and epidermal growth factor receptor overexpression as independent prognostic markers in intracranial ependymoma. *Clin Cancer Res.* 12(7 Pt 1):2070-2079.

[50] Gupta R. K., Sharma M. C., Suri V. et al. (2014). Study of chromosome 9q gain, Notch pathway regulators and Tenascin-C in ependymomas. *J Neurooncol.* 116(2):267-274.

[51] Godfraind C., Kaczmarska J. M., Kocak M. et al. (2014). Distinct disease-risk groups in pediatric supratentorial and posterior fossa ependymoma. *Acta Neuropathol.* 124(2):247-57. doi:10.1007/s00401-012-0981-9.

[52] Suarez-Merino B., Hubank M., Revesz T. et al. (2005). Microarray analysis of pediatric ependymoma identifies a cluster of 112 candidate genes including four transcripts at 22q12.1-q13.3. *Neuro Oncol.* 7(1): 20-31.

[53] Rand V., Prebble E., Ridley L. et al. (2008). Investigation of chromosome 1q reveals differential expression of members of the S100 family in clinical subgroups of intracranial pediatric ependymoma. *Br J Cancer.* 99(7): 1136-1143. doi:10.1038/sj.bjc.6604651.

[54] Lukashova-V. Zangen I., Monoranu C. M. et al. (2007). *Ependymoma gene expression profiles associated with histological subtypes, proliferation, and patient survival.* 113(3):325-337.

[55] Sowar K., Straessle J., Donson A. M. et al. (2006). Predicting which children are at risk for ependymoma relapse. *J Neurooncol.* 78(1):41-46.

[56] Puget S., Grill J., Valent A. et al. (2009). Canditate genes on chromosome 9q33-34 involved in the progression of childhood ependymomas. *J* Clin *Oncol.* 27(11):1884-18892. doi:10.1200/JCO. 2007.15.4195.

[57] Taylor M. D., Poppleton H., Fuller C. et al. (2007). Radial glia cells are candidate stem cells of ependymoma. *Br J Cancer.* 96:6-10.

[58] Korshunov A., Neben K., Wrobel G. et al. (2003). Gene expression patterns in ependymomas correlate with tumor location, grade and patient age. *Am J Pathol.* 163(5):1721-1727.

[59] Patjler K. W., Witt H., Sill M. et al. (2015). Molecular classification of ependymal tumors across all CNS compartment, Histopathological Grades and Age Groups. *Cancer Cell.* 27(5):728-43. doi:10.1016/j.ccell. 2015.04. 002.

[60] Mack S. C., Witt H., Piro R. M. et al. (2014). Epigenomic alterations define lethal CIMP-positive ependymomas of infancy. *Nature.* 506 (7489):445-50. doi:10.1038/nature13108.

[61] Hoffman L. M., Donson A. M., Nakachi I. et al. (2014). Molecular sub-group-specific immunophenotypic changes are associated with outcome in recurrent posterior fossa ependymoma. *Acta Neuropathol.* 127:731-745.

[62] Witt H., Mack S. C., Ryzhova M. et al. (2011). Delineation of two clinically and molecularly distinct subgroups of posterior fossa ependymoma. *Cancer Cell.* 20:143-157.

[63] Korshunov A., Witt H., Hielscher T. et al. (2010). Molecular staging of intracranial ependymoma in children and adults. *J Clin Oncol.* 28(19): 3182-90. doi:10.1200/JCO.2009.27.3359.

[64] Griesinger A. M., Josephson R. J., Donson A. M. et al. (2015). Interleukin-6/STAT3 pathway signaling drives an inflammatory phenotype in Group A ependymoma. *Cancer Immunol Res*. 3(10):1165-1174. doi: 10.1158/2326-6066.CIR-15-0061.

[65] Parker M., Mohankumar K. M., Punchihewa C. et al. (2014). C11 orf 95-RELA fusions drive oncogenic NF-kappa B signaling in ependymoma. *Nature*. 506(7849):451-5.

INDEX

#

A

B

C

D

E

I

K

L

M

N

O

P

Q

R

S

T

U

V

W

X

Y